ALMOST ANOREXIC

Is My (or My Loved One's) Relationship with Food a Problem?

Jennifer J. Thomas, PhD, Harvard Medical School

Jenni Schaefer

HAZELDEN®

Hazelden
Center City, Minnesota 55012
hazelden.org

© 2013 by Harvard University
All rights reserved. Published 2013.
Printed in the United States of America

Library of Congress Cataloging-in-Publication Data

Thomas, Jennifer J.
    Almost anorexic : is my (or my loved one's) relationship with food a problem? / Jennifer J. Thomas, Jenni Schaefer.
        pages cm. — (The almost effect series)
    Summary: "Determine if your eating behaviors are a problem, develop strategies to change unhealthy patterns, and learn when and how to get professional help when needed with this practical, engaging guide to taking care of yourself when you are not a full-blown anorexic. Every day millions of us struggle with eating. We stand at the mirror wondering how we can face the day when we look so fat. We over-exercise. We skip meals, go on fad diets, and scan labels for "fat free." Still, we are never thin enough. Sitting down to a meal feels like facing a battle. Many of us suffer from the symptoms and effects of anorexia, but never address the issue because we don't fully meet the diagnostic criteria. One major study estimates that while 1 in 200 adults have experienced the full anorexia syndrome, as many as 1 in 20 have exhibited at least some of the key symptoms. If this is the case for you, then you may be "almost anorexic." With this groundbreaking book, you can get help for yourself or a loved one. Drawing on case studies and the latest research, eating disorder experts Jennifer Thomas and Jenni Schaefer give you the skills to understand the symptoms of almost anorexia and its place on the spectrum from normal eating behaviors to a full-blown eating disorder, determine if you (or your loved one's) relationship with food is a problem, gain insight on how to intervene with a loved one, discover proven strategies to change unhealthy eating patterns, and learn when and how to get professional help when it's needed"— Provided by publisher.
    ISBN 978-1-61649-444-5 (pbk.) — ISBN 978-1-61649-498-8 (ebook)
    1. 1. Anorexia nervosa—Popular works. 2. Eating disorders—Popular works.
I. Schaefer, Jenni. II. Title.
    RC552.A5T488 2013
    616.85'262--dc233
                                                          2013000690

Editor's notes:

The case examples in this book are composite examples based upon behaviors encountered in the authors' own professional experience. None of the individuals described in this book are based on a specific patient, and all identifying details in the composite examples have been changed to protect the privacy of the people involved.

    This publication is not intended as a substitute for the advice of health care professionals.

17 16 15 14 13   1 2 3 4 5 6

Cover design by Theresa Jaeger Gedig
Interior design and typesetting by Kinne Design

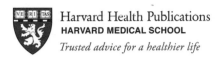

Harvard Health Publications
HARVARD MEDICAL SCHOOL
Trusted advice for a healthier life

The Almost Effect™ **series** presents books written
by Harvard Medical School faculty and other
experts who offer guidance on common behavioral
and physical problems falling in the spectrum between
normal health and a full-blown medical condition.
These are the first publications to help general readers
recognize and address these problems.

For Noah
J.T.

For my nephews
Andrew, Aiden, and Alex
J.S.

contents

List of Tables and Figures

The Almost Effect

I once overheard a mother counseling her grown daughter to avoid dating a man she thought had a drinking problem. The daughter said, "Mom, he's not an alcoholic!" The mother quickly responded, "Well, maybe not, but he *almost* is."

Perhaps you've heard someone, referring to a boss or public figure, say, "I don't like that guy. He's *almost* a psychopath!"

Over the years, I've heard many variations on this theme. The medical literature currently recognizes many problems or syndromes that don't quite meet the standard definition of a medical condition. Although the medical literature has many examples of these syndromes, they are often not well known (except by doctors specializing in that particular area of medicine) or well described (except in highly technical medical research articles). They are what medical professionals often refer to as subclinical and, using the common parlance from the examples above, what we're calling *the almost effect*.

For example:

- Glucose intolerance may or may not always lead to the medical condition of diabetes, but it nonetheless increases your risk of getting diabetes—which then increases your risk of heart attacks, strokes, and many other illnesses.
- Sunburns, especially severe ones, may not always lead to skin cancer, but they always increase your risk of skin cancer, cause immediate pain, and may cause permanent cosmetic issues.
- Pre-hypertension may not always lead to hypertension (high blood pressure), but it increases your risk of getting hypertension, which then increases your risk of heart attacks, strokes, and other illnesses.
- Osteopenia signifies a minor loss of bone that may not always lead to the more significant bone loss called osteoporosis, but it still increases your risk of getting osteoporosis, which then increases your risk of having a pathologic fracture.

Diseases can develop slowly, producing milder symptoms for years before they become full-blown. If you recognize them early, before they become fully developed, and take relatively simple actions, you have a good chance of preventing them from turning into the full-blown disorder. In many instances there are steps you can try at home on your own; this is especially true with the mental and behavioral health disorders.

So, what exactly is the almost effect and why this book? *Almost Anorexic* is one of a series of books by faculty members from Harvard Medical School and other experts. These books are the first to describe in everyday language how to recognize and what to do about some of the most common behavioral and emotional problems that fall within the continuum between normal and full-blown pathology. Since this concept is new and still evolving, we're proposing a new term, *the almost effect*, to describe problems characterized by the following criteria.

The problem

1. falls outside of normal behavior but falls short of meeting the criteria for a particular diagnosis (such as alcoholism, major depression, psychopathy, anorexia nervosa, or substance dependence);

2. is currently causing identifiable issues for individuals and/or others in their lives;

3. may progress to the full-blown condition, meeting accepted diagnostic criteria, but even if it doesn't, still can cause significant suffering;

4. should respond to appropriate interventions when accurately identified.

The Almost Effect

Normal Feelings and Behaviors	The Almost Effect	Condition Meets Diagnostic Criteria for Full-Blown Pathology

All of the books in The Almost Effect™ series make a simple point: Each of these conditions occurs along a spectrum, with normal health and behavior at one end, and the full-blown disorder at the other. Between these two extremes is where the almost effect lies. It is the point at which a person is experiencing real pain and suffering from a condition for which there are solutions—*if* the problem is recognized.

Recognizing the almost effect not only helps a person address real issues now; it also opens the door for change well in advance of the point at which the problem becomes severe. In short, recognizing the almost effect has two primary goals: (1) to alleviate pain and suffering now and (2) to prevent additional problems later.

I am convinced these problems are causing tremendous suffering, and it is my hope that the science-based information in these books can help alleviate this suffering. Readers can find help in the practical self-assessments and advice offered here, and the current research and clinical expertise presented in the series can open opportunities for health care professionals to intervene more effectively.

I hope you find this book helpful. For information about other books in this series, visit www.TheAlmostEffect.com.

Julie Silver, MD
Associate Professor, Harvard Medical School
Chief Editor of Books, Harvard Health Publications

acknowledgments

It takes a lot of people to birth a book. We would like to first thank Julie Silver, MD, and Sid Farrar for your editorial guidance and enthusiasm and Jennifer Hicks and Kristen Casale for your research assistance. This book would surely not exist without your invaluable support. Thanks also to the wonderful staff at both Harvard Health Publications and Hazelden. And to Linda Konner, literary agent for The Almost Effect™ series, we appreciate your making this book a reality as well. Rusty Shelton, thank you for helping us to spread our message of hope far and wide.

To all of our expert book chapter reviewers, we can't thank you enough for sharing your clinical and research insights. You are the best of the best: Ovidio Bermudez, MD; Michael E. Berrett, PhD; Carolyn Costin, LMFT; Sherrie Delinsky, PhD; Kamryn Eddy, PhD; Andrea Hartmann, PhD; Nicole Hawkins, PhD; Abigail Judge, PhD; Walter Kaye, MD; Margo Maine, PhD; Luana Marques, PhD; Beth Hartman McGilley, PhD; Christina Roberto, PhD; Reba Sloan, RD; Sarah St. Germain Smith, PhD; Audrey Tolman, PhD; Ed Tyson, MD; and Jaimie Winkler, RD. We also wish to heartily thank all who provided commentary on drafts of the full manuscript, including Meg

Burton, Lorri Irrgang, Angela Lee, Troy Roness, and Melissa Stone, MA. Although we cannot mention them specifically by name, we would also like to acknowledge the anonymous Harvard faculty peer reviewers who provided important feedback.

Special thanks to all of you who shared your heartfelt stories with us, including Dotsie Bausch, Ragan Chastain, Elijah Corbin, Amanda Olsen, Doris Smeltzer, and Mark Warren, MD, and to you who shared your talents, including artist Emily Wierenga, songwriters Dave Berg and Georgia Middleman ("It's Okay to Be Happy") and Teresa Boaz and Sandy Ramos ("She Blames Herself").

To our friends and family, we could not have finished this book without your undying support and love. With your companionship and laughter, you helped us, throughout the writing process, to mindfully live our message: balance. Dr. Thomas would like to thank her husband Noah Shamosh (for his equanimity), her father Greg Thomas (for his empiricism), and her mother Joanne Coane (for her unconditional love). Jenni would like to thank her parents, Joe and Susan Schaefer, not only for helping her to recover but for encouraging her to pursue a writing career—despite her biochemistry degree! She would also like to recognize Eric Fluhr, Steven and Destiny Schaefer, and Jeffery Schaefer—all of whose continual support made a big difference.

Dr. Thomas would like to thank the organizations that have generously funded her scientific research on almost anorexia, including the Klarman Family Foundation, Hilda and Preston Davis Foundation, and National Institute of Mental Health. She would also like to acknowledge her amazing colleagues at the Massachusetts General Hospital Eating Disorders Clinical and Research Program and McLean Hospital's Klarman Eating Disorders Center. Similarly, Jenni would like to recognize all of her incredible colleagues for both their encouragement and mentorship. Thanks especially to those who helped her along her recovery journey. Jenni also expresses deep thanks to each person who has ever read one of her books. Without people reading her books, she would never have been able to write this one.

Finally, to all of Dr. Thomas's patients and research participants who have honored her with their trust and taught her so much about almost anorexia, thank you. Jenni expresses the same wishes to everyone she has connected with who struggles with disordered eating. Because of you who have shared with us, this book is in your hands.

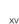

| introduction |

A Touch of Anorexia

"I wish I had just a touch of anorexia."

A young woman whispered this to me after I shared my eating disorder recovery story in her school's auditorium. She had waited patiently to talk with me until most of the crowd had dissipated into the humid evening and I was packing up my guitar.

"Jenni, I never had the problem you had," she continued before I could respond. "I've struggled with *overeating* my entire life." Her eyes darted quickly behind her to confirm that her next statement would be out of public earshot. Then she looked back up at me: "If only I had your willpower, I know I could lose this weight."

• • •

You might have heard someone say this before. Or maybe you've said (or thought) something like it yourself. Countless people want to "eat better" and "lose a few pounds." But, unlike what some may think, anorexia nervosa* is not simply a diet gone wrong, and it has little to do with willpower. Why, then, does a serious, life-threatening illness with one of the highest mortality rates of any psychiatric disorder[1] inspire such cachet?

A superficial response may lie in the current high rates of obesity. With one-third of adult Americans overweight and yet another third obese,[2] the ability to achieve a low body weight by controlling food intake is exceedingly rare. But you've probably never heard people say they wished they had a touch of cancer or depression, two other illnesses that can also lead individuals to eat less and lose weight.

A not-so-obvious—but perhaps more accurate—explanation of anorexia's pseudo-prestige lies in the definition of anorexia nervosa itself. The criteria listed in *DSM-5*, the *Diagnostic and Statistical Manual of Mental Disorders (5th edition)*[3], which health care professionals use to diagnose psychiatric disorders, are quite strictly defined (appendix A). For some, meeting such select criteria can feel like earning a badge of honor. Of course, developing a life-threatening eating disorder is nothing of the sort. The hallmark feature of anorexia nervosa is a significantly low body weight due to self-imposed food restriction. Accompanied by an intense fear of fatness or relentless behavior that interferes with weight gain, anorexia is also characterized by body image disturbance. Not only do individuals with anorexia typically "feel fat" despite being thin; they may also base their self-worth almost entirely on their ability to control their eating and weight.

---

* For brevity's sake, in this book, we will often simply refer to anorexia nervosa as anorexia and to bulimia nervosa as bulimia.

Anorexia is not just a cry for attention; it's a serious mental illness caused by biological, psychological, and environmental factors. A common misconception is that someone with anorexia can "just eat" but is simply choosing not to. Nothing could be further from the truth. Once a person becomes dangerously underweight, powerful psychological and neurobiological changes lock the symptoms in place. Some with anorexia nervosa even begin bingeing and purging, in part, as a result of these physiological changes. Another myth is that anorexia only affects the lives of young white females. Although research suggests that anorexia is more prevalent in females, many males also develop the disorder. Similarly, although the illness typically begins during adolescence with peaks at ages fourteen and eighteen, people of all ages struggle. As a matter of fact, eating disorders do not discriminate by age, gender, culture, ethnicity, sexual orientation, or socioeconomic status.

The truth is that the majority of people with eating disorders do not fulfill anorexia nervosa's diagnostic requirements,[4] nor do the countless others who loathe their bodies and struggle to eat normally. We know from clinical and personal experience that the gray area between normal eating and anorexia nervosa is home to a great deal of pain and suffering for many people. Their lives can be just as out of control, unmanageable, and miserable—if not more so—than those with anorexia. That's why we wrote this book: to identify and provide guidance for people who struggle with forms of disordered eating that are not officially recognized and often go untreated—what some clinicians have termed "diagnostic orphans." We call this once-overlooked category *almost anorexic.*

In the simplest terms, *almost anorexic* describes subclinical levels of eating disorder symptoms. When we say "subclinical," we mean that key symptoms of an illness are present but not in the quantity or severity to meet criteria for an official *DSM-5* diagnosis. (You will see references to *"DSM"* throughout this book. Again, this is a manual that clinicians use to help make diagnoses.) Subclinical illnesses like almost anorexia often sneak below the radar of clinical detection. For example, a formerly heavy man who drops pounds through extremely restrictive eating may have almost anorexia even if he does not have a significantly low weight. Similarly, an underweight woman who does not feel fat or fear gaining weight would have almost anorexia if she feels terrified to relinquish the rigid dietary rules that dominate her life.

Diagnostic criteria are just guidelines, and people whose symptoms don't quite fit those parameters can still suffer. Forget about the key symptoms of anorexia for a minute, and just consider this: to what extent is a preoccupation with eating, shape, and weight impairing your life? If *almost anorexic* seems to describe you or your loved one, we hope that this book will provide help and a real path to healing.

• • •

Who are we anyway? We are two people who know eating disorders—inside and out.

Jennifer J. Thomas, PhD, is an assistant professor of psychology at Harvard Medical School, where her research focuses on enhancing eating disorder diagnostic criteria to better reflect the experience of real patients. Dr. Thomas dedicated her career to eating disorders after spending her teen years as a preprofessional ballet dancer and witnessing firsthand how much the thin ideal can impact young women's self-esteem. Her research studies have received both federal and foundation funding, and she has published over forty articles and chapters, many of which will be described in this book. People who are familiar with Dr. Thomas know that she may love to wear pearls and do research, but she doesn't sit in an ivory tower. As a clinical psychologist in the eating disorder programs at two Harvard teaching hospitals (Massachusetts General Hospital and McLean Hospital), she has evaluated and treated—in both inpatient and outpatient settings—hundreds of individuals of all ages with anorexia nervosa and other officially recognized eating disorders. She is also an active member of several international organizations dedicated to eating disorder research, education, prevention, and treatment.

Jenni Schaefer knows what it's like both to have an eating disorder and to fully recover from one. She has written about her journey in two best-selling books. Happily, Jenni discovered that freedom from food and weight obsessions is so much more than just that. She also learned that getting better means getting your life back. Today, Jenni encourages others to jump into their lives, to follow their true passions, and, most of all, to never give up. A singer/songwriter living in Austin, Texas, Jenni is a regular guest on national radio and television shows and a popular speaker around the globe. Jenni doesn't usually wear pearls; they get in the way of things like ice climbing in Alaska (her favorite place to visit).

Since we have written *Almost Anorexic* together, in this book we will sometimes refer to each other in third person (using "she"). Because we share the same first name, we'll refer to Jennifer Thomas as "Dr. Thomas" and Jenni Schaefer as "Jenni." In reality, almost all of Dr. Thomas's patients and colleagues call her "Jenny." So if you can keep the two of us straight, feel free to mentally replace "Dr. Thomas" with "Jenny" as you read. Jenni's battle with almost anorexia will be highlighted throughout this book, particularly in the "Jenni's Journey" sidebars, written by Jenni herself. Like most people who develop a full-blown eating disorder, she experienced subclinical symptoms first.

Almost Anorexia: Jenni's Story

At four years old, I already heard a negative voice in my head saying, "You're fat. You aren't good enough." I remember wearing a little yellow tutu onstage during a dance recital—feeling fat. The recital was purely for fun, not competition. But I couldn't help but compare my size to the other little girls in my class. In elementary school, I was afraid to eat birthday cake at friends' parties. After trick-or-treating, I carefully saved my Halloween candy in the back of my closet, only to throw it away the following October.

Looking back at my middle school years, I must have had very low self-esteem. I didn't realize it back then, though, because I had gained a false sense of confidence from achievement and status. I remember counting the number of brand-name items in my closet from back-to-school shopping trips. I had one pair of Guess jeans. But Michelle had five. I was chosen to play basketball in sports class, but not for the "A" team. Playing on the "B" team made me feel like I was inadequate in some way. Nothing was ever enough. I was in tier two of the social hierarchy, a great, well-liked group of kids, but not the most popular crowd. On some level, I thought that if only I were thin enough, maybe I would fit in and be okay. During these years, I was also quite confused and worried, not to mention absolutely terrified about puberty and all of the associated body changes. Trying to control my food intake made me feel like I had at least some power over my ever-changing silhouette.

In high school, I tried to control even more. I became consumed with getting perfect grades. I thought I had to get 100 percent on everything. If not, I beat myself up about it. Yes, I sometimes felt like I had failed if I scored even a 99 percent— after all, that was 1 percent of the material that I didn't know! I also began weighing myself. I bought a little blue scale and stood on it every day. (I hid this obsession from my parents and two brothers, none of whom had ever owned such a contraption.) I constantly compared myself to the other girls in my classes to make sure I was the skinniest in the room. Once, my friend Sandi became so frustrated with how I compared my body to hers—complaining that I felt much larger—that she pulled out a measuring tape to prove that I was actually thinner. That still wasn't enough for me.

By the time I graduated from high school and stepped foot onto my college campus, I was almost anorexic.

This is when my eating behaviors took a turn for the worse. All of a sudden my mom wasn't putting dinner on the table each night at 5 o'clock, so it was easy to skip meals. Women in my dorm invited me to the dining hall, but I usually made an excuse because I wanted to eat alone—to study (in an attempt to continue my trend of perfect grades from high school). I tried diet soda for the first time from my roommate's supply in our fridge and was instantly hooked. Why hadn't I thought of

Diet Dr. Pepper as a meal replacement before? I began to drop pounds.

At the time, I didn't realize that the transition from high school to college had been so difficult for me. Now I can see that all of the changes were affecting me more than I knew. Instead of voicing my concerns to others or even acknowledging them to myself, I just stuffed the fears deep inside. I think the more scared I became, the less I ate.

My new college classmates often asked for my secret: "I can fit my hand around your upper arm," one gushed. "How do you stay so thin?"

But when my longtime high school friends noticed this weight loss, they expressed concern. I had always been a normal weight, although thin, prior to starting college. I knew that I had lost weight, but I honestly believed that I was just healthy. I also felt a strange sense of pride about being able to do what some thought impossible—lose weight. And yet I felt intense pressure to maintain my now-smaller size. I fearfully wondered, *How am I going to be able to stay this thin for the rest of my life?* I actually thought about how I might look at age eighty. Could I still be this thin? (Yes, at eighteen years old, I was already worried about how I would look in a nursing home.)

Because my high school friends seemed so worried about me, I finally went to the student health clinic. "Do you eat?" asked the doctor. "Yes," I replied, recalling my binge earlier that week. I had gotten so hungry from the constant self-imposed food restriction that I couldn't stop myself from eating a party-size bag of pretzels. The embarrassment that I felt about my binge eating was so intense that I couldn't possibly reveal the details. Since that was the only question the doctor asked, I received a clean bill of health.

Looking back, I wish people had recognized that my unhealthy eating habits were a sign of a serious problem. I was in a lot of emotional pain, but there wasn't an avenue to get help. I don't blame the people in my life for this. Just as I hid my devotion to the scale, I also kept secret all of my eating behaviors that I knew implicitly were "different" from the way other people ate. Even so, I didn't realize I was struggling until much later. A thick layer of denial and shame almost always accompanies eating-disordered behaviors. Because of this, many people suffer in silence for years.

If my eating disorder symptoms hadn't eventually developed into the specific diagnostic criteria for anorexia nervosa—which happened by the end of my first semester in college—chances are that I never would have taken my illness seriously enough to get help. I might have lived my entire life in a miserable state, expending way too much time, energy, and thought on calorie counting and body loathing. I might have never stopped listening to that voice inside that said, "You aren't enough."

Although it was years after my initial visit to the student health clinic, I gratefully entered treatment for anorexia nervosa at age twenty-two. In therapy, I learned to name that negative voice "Ed," which is an acronym for "eating disorder." I was taught to personify my eating disorder and treat it like a relationship rather than an illness or a condition. Being with Ed was similar in many ways to an abusive marriage. Ed told me that I was worthless and beat me up physically. But I couldn't figure out how to leave "him" (even when I wanted to). The metaphor of Ed was simply a tool I used to separate from the illness and to find my own unique voice and personality. Described thoroughly in my first book, *Life Without Ed*,[5] this externalization technique allowed me to separate from the illness and to make room for my authentic self. In the beginning, a typical conversation with Ed went something like this:

Ed: Your legs are fat.

Jenni: I know.

Ed: You should skip lunch today.

Jenni: Okay.

Throughout recovery, I learned not only to separate from Ed, like the dialogue above shows, but also to disagree with him. Ultimately, with the support of health care professionals, friends, and family, I gained the strength to disobey too. My attitudes and behaviors with food began to improve. In this book, my recovery may appear quick and easy—it will sometimes seem like I got better in a matter of pages (or even within a paragraph). I assure you that the process was not that simple. The real pages in my life took much time and patience.

It's important to note that on my way out of anorexia nervosa, I found myself experiencing almost anorexic symptoms again. This time, almost anorexia meant both that I was getting better and that I still had room to grow. I didn't want to settle for living with almost anorexia when complete freedom could be a reality for me. As before, almost anorexia could have pushed me into full-blown anorexia again or, if not, into full-blown misery. I didn't want either. So, I kept taking steps forward and finally, I "divorced" Ed completely.

• • •

Although Jenni didn't learn about the concept of "Ed" until after she had developed severe anorexia nervosa, she believes it could have been an invaluable tool in the early stages of her illness. That is why, in this book, we introduce the concept, which is used by experts worldwide. Do you have an "Ed" in your head? If so, it can be important to think about yourself as separate from it. You don't have to be defined by your problem. To help distinguish yourself from the negative voice in your head, you might experiment with using the Ed metaphor. Some people we know find the metaphor useful, but they change the name from "Ed" to something that rings more true for them. For example, some use the name "Rex" for ano-*rex*-ia. Others view the voice as a female and thus refer to their eating disorders as "Ana" or "Mia," which are short for *ana*-rexia and buli-*mia*, respectively. It doesn't matter what you name that voice or even if you decide to name it at all. What is significant is that you realize disordered eating does not have to define you. But remember that treating your eating disorder like a relationship is just a metaphor—a tool that may help you. In her second book, *Goodbye Ed, Hello Me*, Jenni clarified, "Of course, my eating disorder was never really a guy named Ed who followed me around night and day, but it sure felt like it. Ed stood for a collection of beliefs I had learned since I was born. Unlike other recovery models, I learned that Ed was not an aspect of my authentic self, so my goal was always to separate from him. Different recovery models and tools work better for different people."[6] If the externalization technique works for you, keep in mind that separating from your illness is not about blaming the eating disorder: *Ed made me do it*. Rather, the purpose of separating from Ed is to help yourself become accountable for how you respond to him.

You might notice that Ed is already starting to talk to you about this book and the almost anorexia concept, saying things like "You are such a failure at your eating disorder because you don't meet anorexia criteria," or "Way to go. If you keep this up, you just might reach full-fledged anorexia soon," as if the anorexic label were some kind of trophy. Or maybe Ed is just telling you that we don't have any idea what we are talking about! We wouldn't be surprised. Ed's role is to get you to focus on anything but getting better.

It's Not Black and White

Most people think that you either have anorexia or you don't, as depicted in Figure 1.

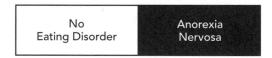

Figure 1.

The Dichotomy Model of Anorexia Nervosa

But that is not what the research shows. Eating disorders are far more complex than this simple diagram implies. The officially recognized *DSM-5* feeding and eating disorders are *anorexia nervosa, bulimia nervosa* (binge eating with compensatory behaviors), *binge eating disorder* (binge eating without compensatory behaviors), *avoidant/restrictive food intake disorder* (inadequate nutritional intake in the absence of body image concerns), *pica* (repeated consumption of nonfood items such as chalk), and *rumination disorder* (bringing food back up into one's mouth in order to re-chew or re-swallow it). In *DSM-5*, each of these eating disorders has its own set of specific criteria that can rule someone in or out of the diagnosis. See appendix A for details. In this book, the eating disorders (anorexia, bulimia, and binge eating disorder) will be discussed whereas the feeding disorders (avoidant/restrictive food intake disorder, pica, and rumination disorder) will not.

In our experience, individuals with disordered eating usually view themselves as part of an unspoken hierarchy. One patient described it like this: "Anorexia is like Saks [Fifth Avenue], bulimia is Target, and binge eating disorder is Wal-Mart."[7] Indeed, anorexia nervosa has a sought-after status that people often try to move toward regardless of the nature of their specific problems with food and weight. Using this line of warped thinking, almost anorexia might be seen as a thrift store or garage sale. But this model is both flawed and damaging. We have seen that people with almost anorexia sometimes feel worse than those who actually have anorexia nervosa, because those with almost anorexia assume that they are not "sick enough" to deserve help and so, sadly, never seek it.

Because we believe that most individuals with disordered eating can relate to an "anorexic mind-set" that prioritizes extreme thinness and dietary restriction, we have called this book *Almost Anorexic* instead of *Almost an Eating Disorder.* But we will cover the broad range of abnormal behaviors that exist with food and weight—not just food restriction and weight loss. Within this book, we will talk about bingeing and purging behaviors as well as negative body image. As you will see, in Jenni's story among others, there are many levels to almost anorexia. It's also important to remember that eating-disordered behaviors might look different, and body shapes and sizes may vary, but a similar pain goes on inside.

You might have noticed that we use the term *almost anorexic* as an adjective rather than a noun. We would never label someone who suffers as being *an almost anorexic*. Rather, a person might struggle with almost anorexic thoughts and behaviors. Labeling is not our intent. We describe almost anorexic as a vehicle for people like you or your loved one to get much-needed help.

For simplicity's sake, we address this book primarily to individuals who might have almost anorexia. Of course, we are also writing this book for loved ones and for professionals who treat eating disorders, which is actually another reason we chose this specific format. In numerous treatment programs, Jenni's previous books, which are also addressed to the sufferer, have been required reading both for staff and for patients' families. This is because the books provide a novel window into the mind of someone who experiences disordered eating. If you are worried about a loved one, *Almost Anorexic* will provide another source of unique and helpful insights. You will get a firsthand view of what it is like to be trapped inside almost anorexia.

We have made every effort to avoid providing details that individuals struggling with almost anorexia might find "triggering." In other words, we don't want this book to be used as a "how-to guide" for developing an eating disorder. Patients' diet tips and preferred brand of laxatives will not be discussed. Of course, some specifics are necessary in order for you to make a decision about whether you (or your loved one) might have almost anorexia. You can think about it this way: if this book is "triggering," that may be important diagnostic information.

If just reading about eating, weight, and shape causes someone distress, that individual may fall into the almost anorexic group or even have a full-blown eating disorder.

While part 1 of this book describes almost anorexia in greater detail, including key symptoms, part 2 offers solutions based on empirical research, Dr. Thomas's clinical practice, and Jenni's personal experience. We have included self-help exercises, as well as advice on identifying treatment resources.

We have tried to jam-pack this book with information without making it feel overwhelming. To do this, we have broken each chapter into numerous sections with subheadings. When Jenni was sick with Ed screaming in her ear, she found it difficult to concentrate on reading a lot of material at once. Relating to her experience, you might prefer to read only a section or two of this book at a time. Or you might even choose to skip certain sections. (Maybe you really don't want to know any more about the *DSM*!) And that's okay. We wrote this book so that you can take from it what you find helpful and not worry about the rest. We do hope you will keep reading, so that you can begin to tackle any problems you might have with food and weight.

As Jenni once did, you might sometimes wonder, as you review self-help strategies, *Will this really work?* Jenni was surprised when Dr. Thomas told her that many of the ideas she had relied on in her own recovery were backed by science. So to answer the question, research says yes. Although different strategies work for different people, one thing is certain: something will work for you.

Part 1

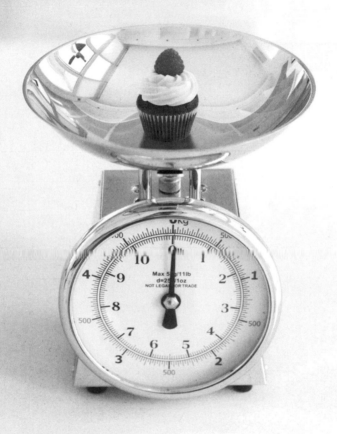

Getting to Know the Ed
in Your Head

1

What Is Almost Anorexia?

This might surprise you, but anorexic symptoms lie on a continuum with normal eating.[1] On the left end (figure 2), people eat in a balanced way and don't worry much about their weight. Those to the far right are diagnosed with anorexia nervosa and other officially recognized eating disorders.

Figure 2.
Anorexic Continuum

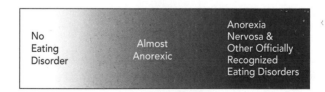

The people in the middle—the gray area—don't have an officially recognized eating disorder, yet they don't eat normally either. They may feel preoccupied with their body image, go on crash diets, and consider drastic weight-loss strategies. They may meet some, but not all, criteria for anorexia, bulimia, or binge eating disorder. Many of these people—suffering immensely—have almost anorexia. This was true for a young woman we'll call Taylor.

Taylor

"I want a body just like yours—only fifteen pounds lighter." When Taylor heard these words coming from her client Kelly, she did all that she could to not break down and cry right in the middle of that weight-training session. At age thirty, Taylor was a successful personal trainer, and her community considered her an expert on wellness. But inside, she felt like a fraud. She helped clients daily to achieve their fitness goals but couldn't seem to help herself. Her mounting guilt only seemed to make her own problem with food and weight worse.

As far back as she could remember Taylor had been in a close—albeit tumultuous—relationship with food. Early on, she liked reading about food in magazines, experimenting with new recipes, and enjoying occasional treats with family and friends. When she was eighteen, her relationship with food took a turn during short stints at various colleges. As she became more worried and anxious about what she wanted to be "when she grew up," she turned to food to cope. Taylor felt like society expected her to get a degree, and while she certainly had the brains for it, she didn't have the desire. A free spirit, Taylor never loved being in the classroom. After sending in her application for yet one more university, she distinctly remembers rushing back to her apartment and eating an entire jar of peanut butter followed by a whole loaf of bread. Horrified, Taylor wondered, *What is wrong with me? Why can't I stop eating?* She felt ashamed and decided to put a tighter rein on her diet.

She made a mental note, *No more peanut butter or bread allowed in the apartment. Fruits and vegetables only.* But the more she restricted her diet, the more out of control her eating became. Although Taylor only binged every few weeks, the amount of pain, discomfort, and shame that she felt as a result was enough to last all month long. And even when she wasn't bingeing, her eating was often sporadic and unplanned. In the evening, she sometimes found herself going to the apartment complex's vending machine to buy snacks like popcorn and pretzels that she would nibble on while watching television. Although the amount each time was no more than a handful, she was terrified that the calories would add up. In her early twenties, Taylor gained a noticeable amount of weight and felt uncomfortable in her body for the first time in her life. She started working out more—staying longer at the gym each day. When she looked in the mirror, Taylor saw a "fat" person, even though her weight was just slightly above normal for her height.

Blaming her eating patterns entirely on the pursuit of a college degree, she finally decided to quit and follow her true passion. She had always wanted to work in the health and wellness area to help other people. So, at age twenty-five, she began earning certifications in fitness areas, including yoga, Pilates, aerobics, and personal training. She also attended workshops all over the country to learn about alternative approaches to health, with a particular interest in nutrition.

Taylor thought that each new approach to wellness might bring balance to her life. When she received emails on opportunities to learn about both colonics and juice cleansing, she signed up right away. In the beginning, colonics—a process of infusing water into the colon in an effort to cleanse and flush—seemed to be the perfect solution to her binges. *I can flush all of that peanut butter right out of my system*, she thought. But, after only a few weeks, she realized that the colonics weren't working. Her out-of-control eating continued—and seemed to get worse. So she decided to devote more of her efforts to juice cleansing (drinking liquefied fruits and vegetables). Again, at the start, this made her feel like she was somehow making up for her binges, and this time, she even felt thinner. She even received compliments from family, friends, and clients, including Kelly.

In reality, Taylor wasn't losing weight. She was just dehydrated. Meanwhile, she lacked energy, had trouble concentrating, and felt just plain miserable. When her weight eventually started creeping up again, she decided to talk with a fellow personal trainer at the gym, who looked at Taylor and, thinking that she looked fine, simply handed her a piece of paper detailing yet another "new and improved" approach to life. Taylor tossed the paper in the trash and immediately went to the store to buy a jar of peanut butter.

Symptoms of Almost Anorexia

Instead of dismissing Taylor's concerns, what if the trainer had asked her some key questions about her relationship with food and weight? Taylor's answers would have quickly revealed that her struggles placed her along the anorexic continuum.

The close relationship between almost anorexia and other officially recognized eating disorders, which is illustrated in the Anorexic Web we created, often goes unnoticed.

Figure 3.
Anorexic Web

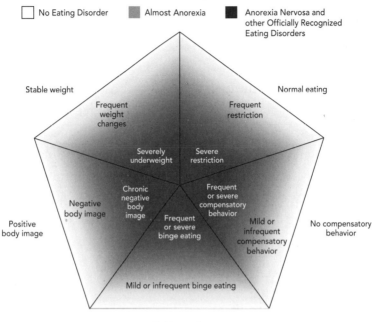

With the five sides of the web each representing varying degrees of eating disorder symptoms, the increasingly darker shading illustrates the progression from no eating disorder (white) to almost anorexia (gray) to anorexia nervosa and other officially recognized eating disorders (black). The Anorexic Web is simply a tool to help you better visualize the complexity of eating disorders—with all of the diverse possible combinations of symptoms—and to guide you in determining where you might fit in. The symptoms of almost anorexia discussed here are also the warning signs to look for if you are concerned about a loved one.

People with anorexia, bulimia, and binge eating disorder generally fall inside the center of the web (experiencing at least two symptoms in the black zone) while those who do not struggle typically fall outside of the web altogether. In contrast, individuals with almost anorexia usually exhibit a consistent pattern of behaviors that fall within the gray zone, between an officially recognized eating disorder and no eating disorder at all. Most people with almost anorexia will experience at least two of the symptoms depicted in gray, but eating disorders are far too complex to give hard and fast rules. For example, certain people with almost anorexia might have one symptom that falls in the black zone and none in the gray zone. Likewise, a person with no eating disorder might at times experience one symptom in the gray area. To avoid any confusion, what really matters is this: if you tend to live your life inside the web rather than outside it, you might have almost anorexia. Taylor was certainly living her life inside the web, struggling with all five symptoms in the gray zone. The more symptoms a person has in the center of the web, the more likely it is that he or she has anorexia, bulimia, or binge eating disorder. Let's take a closer look at the five gray-zone symptoms to help illustrate the difference between almost anorexia and officially recognized eating disorders. You might want to log your answers to the coinciding five questions in a journal.

Frequent Weight Changes

Does your weight shift due to intentional attempts to drop pounds? An essential feature of anorexia nervosa is being extremely underweight. Of course, not all individuals who are underweight have anorexia, but someone cannot be diagnosed with the disorder without a significantly low weight. Because the diagnosis depends on an individual's actual weight rather than his or her degree of weight loss, someone could lose 10, 20, or even 100 pounds using unhealthy behaviors and would not officially have anorexia unless the final number on the scale fell within the underweight range. Yet drastic intentional weight loss or frequent weight changes like Taylor's are a red flag for almost anorexia. Because people without eating disorders usually maintain a relatively stable weight or slowly gain weight as they get older, frequent weight changes often go hand in hand with other symptoms in the gray zone.

Frequent Restriction

Do you regularly restrict food by amount or variety? People with anorexia nervosa severely limit the number of calories they eat. On the flip side, those without eating disorders typically eat when they are hungry, stop when they are full, and allow themselves to enjoy occasional treats. Normal eating like this means that you don't have to eat all of the treats at once—you can choose to leave some for later. In this way, mild restriction is considered a part of normal eating. If your doctor has encouraged you to drop pounds to prevent the onset or exacerbation of an obesity-related medical condition, following a structured eating plan to make small, sensible changes may preserve your good health. However, examples of food restriction that might be considered almost anorexic include attempts to follow rigid dietary rules like only eating at specific times (such as no eating after 7 p.m.), only eating a preset small number of calories (such as less than 1,000) per day, or only eating a limited number of "safe" foods (no white sugar or flour, for example).[2]

Breaking these rules typically leads to extreme guilt. American journalist Katie Couric, who battled bulimia from her late teens to early twenties, described "feeling that if you eat one thing that's wrong, you're full of self-loathing and then you punish yourself, whether it's one cookie or a stick of gum that isn't sugarless. . . . I would sometimes beat myself up for that."[3]

While restricting might be easy to observe in some cases, in others it isn't. Some people with almost anorexia might eat normally around other people but eat very little, or nothing at all, when alone. A telltale sign of Taylor's restricting behavior was that she only kept certain types of food—just fruits and vegetables—in her home. Food restriction often manifests as limiting variety. In our society where such an abundant range of food is available—with more and more choices continually added—there also seems to be an ever-increasing list of ways for people to decrease their own personal food options. (Isn't that ironic?)

Mild or Infrequent Compensatory Behaviors

Do you ever try to "make up for" calories consumed? Frequent or severe compensatory behavior is a defining feature of anorexia nervosa (binge/purge type)* and bulimia nervosa. Compensatory behaviors include purging (self-induced vomiting; inappropriate use of laxatives, medications, enemas, or diuretics) and nonpurging (fasting or excessive exercise) forms. If you are concerned that a loved one may be vomiting, evidence might include calluses on the knuckles and "chipmunk cheeks" or

---

* *DSM-5* recognizes two subtypes of anorexia nervosa: restricting type (in which individuals maintain their low weight by restricting their calorie intake) and binge/ purge type (in which individuals alternate periods of restricting with periods of bingeing and/or purging).

swollen salivary glands. Although different in form, all compensatory behaviors are intended to compensate for, or "get rid of," food that has already been eaten. Most attempts to compensate are just that—attempts. They are not effective for long-term weight loss. Individuals with almost anorexia may engage in these behaviors infrequently (a bulimia diagnosis requires weekly purging) or use milder forms of compensatory behaviors, as Taylor did, including juice fasts, colonics, or cleanses. They also might exercise in a moderate but obligatory —"I have to no matter what"—kind of way. Even though moderate exercise can be enjoyable and healthy, huffing and puffing on the elliptical machine until you have burned the exact amount of calories you just consumed in your last meal or binge is an eating-disordered compensatory behavior. Another example of mild purging might be vomiting "just a little bit" after a meal that makes you feel overly full, rather than trying to throw up the entire meal. But make no mistake: self-induced vomiting is still self-induced vomiting.

Mild or Infrequent Binge Eating

Do you ever eat large amounts of food while feeling out of control? You may be surprised to learn that eating too much can be a symptom of anorexia, even though most people associate the disorder with eating too little. However, a diagnosis of anorexia nervosa (binge/purge type), bulimia nervosa, or binge eating disorder actually requires frequent bingeing. Binge eating involves consuming a large amount of food (for example, two boxes of cereal with milk, a whole large pizza, or all of this plus more) in a short period of time (usually less than two hours). Signs that your loved one might be bingeing include the disappearance of large amounts of food as well as an abundance of food wrappers in the trash can. Because we all overeat once in a while, a true binge also requires a sense of loss of control. Describing bingeing to her therapist, Jenni used to say, "I feel like my body is literally being taken over by something that only cares about eating more and more food. Nothing else matters." Many people who binge will describe a feeling of being "possessed" like this. Of course, they are not truly possessed, but the loss of control makes it feel that way. Looking back, Jenni can see clearly that her bingeing was usually a direct result of restricting. Even though she had lost touch with feelings of physical hunger much of the time, her body was starving for food and would do anything to get it. Clearly, bingeing is much different from enjoying a second helping of pumpkin pie on Thanksgiving or a mint chip ice-cream cone on a hot summer day, both of which are examples of normal eating. In almost anorexia, binges may be infrequent (that is, less than once a week), like Taylor's, or not objectively large. For example, a man with almost anorexia might eat that same amount of pumpkin pie or ice cream but feel like he has lost control while doing it. He then feels guilty, believing that he has eaten a huge amount of food (even though he hasn't) and plans a long run the next morning to make up for it. Alternatively, a pattern of continuously eating small amounts of food over a long period of time is called grazing. Taylor, for example, sometimes grazed while watching television.

Negative Body Image

Does negative body image interfere with living your life to the fullest? Anorexia and bulimia are typically characterized by chronic negative body image. Individuals with anorexia are terrified of gaining weight, and those with bulimia and binge eating disorder often view weight and shape as a major component of self-worth. People with these disorders often will say that they "hate" their bodies. This level of disgust would fall within the black zone of the Anorexic Web. Because very few people look like fashion models or bodybuilders, feeling physically inadequate once in a while does not make you almost anorexic. In fact, experts coined the term "normative discontent" nearly thirty years ago to describe the low-level body dissatisfaction that plagues modern women.[4] A person with a positive body image will still experience this normative discontent at times (Dr. Thomas was not very happy to discover her first gray hair at age twenty-five!) However, if you often feel fat, hop on and off your bathroom scale multiple times per day, or refuse to go to the beach because you are afraid to wear a swimsuit in public, your body image might fall within the gray zone of the web. Obviously, Taylor was becoming increasingly dissatisfied with her weight. At certain points during Jenni's struggle, she did not hate her body, but her identity was so wrapped around staying small that fears about gaining weight unquestionably disrupted her life.

• • •

Do your answers to these five questions lead you to believe that you might have almost anorexia? If your attitudes and behaviors fall within the gray or black zones on the Anorexic Web, we recommend that you use the following tool to further assess your risk.

Are You Almost Anorexic?

Clinical psychologist David Garner and psychiatrist Paul Garfinkel developed the Eating Attitudes Test (EAT-26) over three decades ago,[5] and it is still the most widely used eating disorder screening measure today. This test was designed for use as part of a two-stage screening process. In stage 1, individuals take a three-step questionnaire independently. If they score above the cutoff in step 1, have a low body mass index (BMI, step 2), or exhibit any disordered-eating behaviors in step 3, then they advance to stage 2, where they are interviewed by a clinician to determine whether they meet criteria for a specific eating disorder. In other words, the EAT-26 can't tell you for sure whether you have an eating disorder—only a qualified health professional can do that. However, the test can tell you if your concerns about eating and weight are higher than most people's and if you would benefit from a professional evaluation.

Because hand-scoring the EAT-26 takes time, researchers and clinicians like Dr. Thomas generally use a computer program for calculations. For instructions on taking the test online, visit www.eat-26.com. However, if you just love math and would prefer to crunch numbers yourself, use table 1 (which follows) to fill in your responses or record your responses in a notebook. Refer to appendix B for scoring instructions. Whether you take the test online or by hand, be sure to read the important score interpretation details that follow.

Before you begin, it is important to discuss step 2—BMI. If determining this number were not a component of the EAT-26, we would not have included the idea in this book. Our reluctance to include this step is due to the fact that Ed (or whatever you've named your negative voice regarding your relationship with food) loves to use BMI against people. So, before determining yours, we'd like to make two critical points. First, if you can rule yourself into the almost anorexia category by using steps 1 and 3, and Ed is chomping at the bit to get ahold of yet another number that he can use to torture you, then stop. Calculating your BMI may feel too triggering right now, and that's okay. But remember what we said about triggers. If crunching numbers is a scary thought, this gives you important diagnostic information about a potentially unhealthy attitude you may have toward weight and shape. Second, if you already realize that you are underweight, and you know Ed will use step 2 to cheer on your restricting, there is no need to give him more ammunition—just skip it and move on.

What Does My Score Mean?

Step 1: Attitudes. If your total score is 20 or greater (see appendix B) but you do not meet the diagnostic criteria for anorexia, bulimia, or binge eating disorder (see appendix A), then you may have almost anorexia. While the usual cutoff used by professionals is 20, some studies indicate that a score of just 10 or 11 might signal a problem with eating.[6] All in all, there is no magic number revealing who does and doesn't have an eating disorder. The EAT-26 is simply meant to provide some basic guidelines and is very helpful in doing just that.

Step 2: Body Weight. If you are over age eighteen, your BMI falls above 17.5 but below 18.5 kg/m², and you are actively restricting your intake to stay this size, you may have almost anorexia. While a BMI below 17.5 in an adult is consistent with anorexia nervosa, most individuals will need to restrict their food intake substantially to maintain a long-term BMI less than 18.5.

Table 1.

Eating Attitudes Test (EAT-26)

INSTRUCTIONS: This screening measure helps you determine whether you might have an eating disorder that needs professional attention. It is not designed to diagnose an eating disorder or take the place of a professional consultation. Please fill out the form below as accurately, honestly, and completely as possible. There are no right or wrong answers.

STEP 1: ATTITUDES

Please check a response for the following statements.	Always	Usually	Often	Sometimes	Rarely	Never
1. I am terrified about being overweight.						
2. I avoid eating when I am hungry.						
3. I find myself preoccupied with food.						
4. I have gone on eating binges where I feel that I may not be able to stop.						
5. I cut my food into small pieces.						
6. I am aware of the calorie content of foods that I eat.						
7. I particularly avoid food with a high carbohydrate content (e.g., bread, rice, etc.).						
8. I feel that others would prefer if I ate more.						
9. I vomit after I have eaten.						
10. I feel guilty after eating.						

11.	I am preoccupied with a desire to be thinner.				
12.	I think about burning up calories when I exercise.				
13.	Other people think that I am too thin.				
14.	I am preoccupied with the thought of having fat on my body.				
15.	I take longer than others to eat my meals.				
16.	I avoid eating foods with sugar in them.				
17.	I eat diet foods.				
18.	I feel that food controls my life.				
19.	I display self-control around food.				
20.	I feel that others pressure me to eat.				
21.	I give too much time and thought to food.				
22.	I feel uncomfortable after eating sweets.				
23.	I engage in dieting behavior.				
24.	I like my stomach to be empty.				
25.	I have the impulse to vomit after meals.				
26.	I enjoy trying new rich foods.				

CONTINUED ON NEXT PAGE

STEP 2: BODY WEIGHT

Indicate your height (in feet and inches) and your weight (in pounds).

Height: _____

Weight: _____

STEP 3: BEHAVIORS

In the past 6 months, have you . . . :	Never	Once a month or less	2 to 3 times a month	Once a week	2 to 6 times a week	Once a day or more
A. Gone on eating binges where you felt you might not be able to stop? *(Binges are defined as eating much more than most people would under the same circumstances and feeling that eating is out of control.)*						
B. Ever made yourself sick (vomited) to control your shape or weight?						
C. Ever used laxatives, diet pills, or diuretics (water pills) to control your weight?						
D. Exercised more than 60 minutes a day to lose or control your weight?						
E. Lost 20 pounds or more in the past 6 months?		Yes			No	

Note: The EAT-26 has been reproduced with permission. You can also complete it online at www.eat-26.com.

If your BMI falls in the range of normal (18.5–24.9), over-weight (25.0–29.9), or obese (30.0 and above), and you do not meet diagnostic criteria for bulimia or binge eating disorder, you may still have almost anorexia if you score above the cutoff in step 1 or engage in any disordered-eating behaviors in step 3. If you are under age eighteen, see appendix B for interpreting your BMI.

Because the BMI formula does not distinguish between fat mass and fat-free mass like muscle and bone, a number in the overweight or even the obese range does not automatically mean that you have excess body fat. When Miami Heat basketball star Shaquille O'Neal learned that his BMI of 31.6 put him in the obese category, he famously told the Associated Press, "I've read that same formula, but as an athlete, I'm classified as phenomenal. You can look it up."[7] We totally agree.

Step 3: Behaviors. If you scored any points in this section but do not meet diagnostic criteria for anorexia, bulimia, or binge eating disorder, you may fall into the almost anorexic category.

It Comes Down to This

If you scored a 20 or above in step 1, are maintaining a BMI less than 18.5 (adults) by actively restricting your food intake, or received any points in step 3, we recommend that you seek a professional evaluation. Each of these findings alone is an important indicator of almost anorexia or an officially recognized eating disorder. You don't need to meet all three criteria.

In contrast, if the EAT-26 does not indicate that you have a problem but you feel like food and weight control your life, get help. The test sometimes misses people, especially those who have just two or three symptoms in the gray zone of the

Anorexic Web. Also, keep in mind that the EAT-26 may fail to detect eating disorders in certain groups: among young people who cannot fully articulate their symptoms; in Asian cultures where patients with anorexia do not always endorse a fear of weight gain; or during the honeymoon phase of the illness, when the costs of the disorder are minimized or denied.

How Would Taylor Score on the EAT-26?

Taylor would have scored around an 18—just below the cutoff. Of course, you know from reading her story that Taylor does,

Jenni's Journey

"You don't binge enough," Ed said, as I was checking out a website about eating disorder signs and symptoms. *"And there is no way that you are thin enough to have a real problem,"* he continued. One of Ed's go-to strategies was to tell me that I was okay—even healthier than other people—and to use anything at all to prove his point. With the EAT-26, Ed would have said that I didn't score high enough in step 1—regardless of the number. Similarly, my BMI and disordered-eating behaviors fluctuated so much during the course of my illness that I might have scored in the unhealthy range on steps 2 and 3 some days, but not others. Most people cross over from one symptom or diagnosis to another during the course of their struggle. Ed will attempt to use definitions and tests to confuse you. Remember, we included the EAT-26 in this book purely as a way to rule yourself in, *not* out. If you score in the unhealthy range, the test indicates that you might have almost anorexia or an officially recognized eating disorder. But if you score in the healthy range and still feel that a preoccupation with food and weight is disrupting your life, please don't let a number keep you from getting help.

in fact, have almost anorexia. Her score turned out this way because Taylor would have answered "Usually" or "Often" to most of the questions from 1 to 25, rather than "Always." She would certainly respond to some items as "Always," including 11 (I am preoccupied with a desire to be thinner) and 18 (I feel that food controls my life) but not enough to raise her score to 20. Interestingly, part of the reason that Taylor might not mark as many "Always" has to do with her career in the wellness field. She knows what the "correct" answer should be, so she leans that way even when it goes against how she feels. In step 2, the EAT-26 would have indicated that her weight had always been in the normal range or slightly above. In step 3, Taylor would not have scored any points even though she experiences both bingeing and weight fluctuation. She never lost twenty pounds in six months, and she wouldn't report bingeing two to three times per month. Thus, even though Taylor was exhibiting many distressing eating disorder symptoms, the EAT-26 would not have identified a problem. But people like Taylor deserve help.

2

Becoming Almost Anorexic

Not everyone who worries about what he or she eats and weighs has a problem with food. And not all attempts to eat healthfully are bad. But crossing the fine line from normal eating to almost anorexia—even just a little—can be a big problem. When food and weight begin to consume your life, joy is often what gets cut out to make room for all of that obsessing. Emma knows this all too well.

Emma

Upon graduating from a prestigious Chicago arts college, twenty-two-year-old Emma couldn't wait to move to California with her boyfriend, Sean, who had just been accepted to law school. A shy and bookish Midwestern native, Emma saw her relocation as the perfect opportunity to reinvent herself. She approached the Los Angeles lifestyle with zeal—adding blond highlights to her chestnut brown hair, ordering vegan wraps at hipster cafés, and interviewing for countless jobs in her chosen field of photography. But within a few weeks, she found herself second-guessing the move. Despite her impeccable résumé, the recession meant fewer employment opportunities. Back home she had a close-knit group of girlfriends, but now she found it difficult to meet new people without the predictable structure of school. Trying to hide her disappointment from Sean, Emma took a part-time retail job at a Santa Monica boutique and re-focused her energies on setting up their new apartment.

Still on a student budget, she snapped up free but mis-matched dinnerware online and started eating from the only matching cup and bowl set. She didn't realize how important this ritual had become until one morning she bubbled up with irritation to see *her* cup, coffee-stained from Sean's all-nighter, lying dirty in the sink. Exasperated, she skipped breakfast. With Sean spending more and more evenings at the law library, their romantic evenings cooking over a bottle of wine dissipated into Emma microwaving steamed vegetables to eat alone in front of the television.

Although Emma considered herself lucky to be employed, she knew she didn't fit in with the other salesgirls at the boutique. The more she told them about her dream of doing photo shoots for national magazines, the more they questioned her commitment to sales. The only thing they complimented was her dietary restraint, calling her "tiny Emma" and marvel-ing at her "super-healthy" lunches of carrot straws and hummus. Never having considered herself particularly thin, Emma stepped on the scale at home one night and was surprised to see that she had lost five pounds from her 5'2" frame since leaving Chicago. The weight loss hadn't been intentional, yet gaining recognition for something—anything—after weeks of unsuccessful job searching, felt absolutely intoxicating to her. Determined to be worthy of her newfound "health nut" moniker, Emma added new rules to her daily regime. She began eliminating snacks, measuring portions, and pushing mealtimes later in the day. When Sean took Emma out for Thai food to celebrate acing his first midterm, Emma vetoed the first restaurant in disgust because it didn't serve brown rice. Sean was impressed with her self-control and happily identified a more health-conscious restaurant where Emma could avoid white carbohydrates.

A welcome side effect of Emma's food restriction was the emotional numbness it provided. Although she had previously characterized herself as pensive and empathic—"crying at the drop of a hat," her mom used to say—she felt increasingly anesthetized to her failed job search and growing emotional distance from Sean. The constant lump in her throat and knot in her stomach were replaced with a new sense of safety and calm.

Her preoccupation with food, on the other hand, was maddening. Her valiant mental efforts did nothing to push away negative thoughts about the minutiae of her diet that bombarded her every moment. *Did I serve myself too many almonds at breakfast? I know I counted them twice. . . . Can I wait until 3 p.m. to eat lunch? If I eat too early, what will I do if I get hungry again and it's not time for dinner? . . . Should I have just one square of chocolate with dinner tonight? If I have one, will I be able to stop?* On some level, she worried that a number of her food rules were irrational—like eating even numbers of foods (eight raisins rather than seven, for example) and eating clockwise around her plate. But Emma felt compelled to follow them.

By the end of the fall, she had lost more weight and her period was intermittent. She couldn't remember the last time she had kissed Sean. Truth be told, she didn't feel very interested in much of anything. Except maybe food. When Sean broke up with her after finals, she had the surreal sensation that she was watching a scene from a movie. She knew that she should feel sad, but she felt nothing. As he admitted guiltily that he had met another woman—someone more "fun"—she wondered absentmindedly whether she had put too much olive oil in their stir-fry earlier that evening.

When Emma arrived at the O'Hare airport baggage claim, her father gasped at her gaunt appearance. "Wow, Emma, you look . . ." her father trailed off. Emma's face burned. "I know." Her father insisted that Emma see her primary care doctor for a checkup and then accompanied her to an appointment the next day.

Emma hopped off the scale and looked at the doctor expectantly as he made a quick note. "OSFED—weight not significantly low," she discreetly read. Because she wasn't aware that OSFED stood for other specified feeding and eating disorders, Emma concluded, *I guess I'm not anorexic after all.* She was surprised at her disappointment.

The Secret World of OSFED

Despite all of the media attention it receives, anorexia nervosa is by far the least common eating disorder. There are many more people who, like Emma, fall in the "almost" category of the anorexic continuum (figure 2). But when was the last time you saw a television story or read a news article about someone overcoming almost anorexia? Probably never. This is not because people don't recover. They do. It's because the illness in its various forms hides in our society.

Other specified feeding and eating disorders, known as OSFED, is a catchall category that includes a wide range of eating disturbances that cause distress and impairment but do not meet the specific criteria for anorexia, bulimia, or binge eating disorder. The majority of individuals with almost anorexia would fall into the OSFED category, but a significant minority would not. Although OSFED is listed as a diagnosis in *DSM-5*, it is not considered an "officially recognized" eating disorder, because it does not have a set of specific diagnostic criteria. Instead it has a list of example OSFED subtypes. There are actually no specific exclusion criteria for OSFED, which requires only that the subclinical eating disturbance results in functional impairment, and that can be difficult to define. Thus the line is very fuzzy between who has OSFED, which denotes a more severe form of almost anorexia, and who has almost anorexia but not OSFED. In this book, you will meet people who fall into both categories.

If this isn't the first book you've read on eating disorders, you may have heard OSFED previously referred to as eating disorder not otherwise specified or EDNOS, the name of this category in previous versions of the *DSM*. People used to complain that the name EDNOS was too long and nonspecific. We realize that the new name is no better, but we are just the messengers! Describing confusion over the EDNOS acronym, clinical dietitian Jillian Lampert told us, "A client once asked me, 'Why should I get help? I don't have a serious problem. I have EDNOS, remember?' Curiously, I asked her what she thought EDNOS meant, to which she replied quickly, 'It means eating disorder not *of severity*!' I was stunned and saddened by the clinical sounding but highly inaccurate definition that was so powerfully convincing her she was unworthy of help."[1] Because most research studies of subclinical eating disorders have focused on EDNOS (eating disorders not *otherwise specified*), you will see the terms EDNOS and OSFED several times throughout this book. You will also see that all subclinical eating disorders—whatever the acronym—are truly worthy of help.

Figure 4.
Anorexic Continuum with OSFED

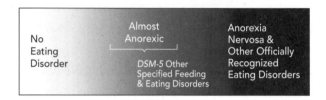

There are five OSFED subtypes, and—as we mentioned above—none of them are considered officially recognized eating disorders. Again, this is because these conditions were identified more recently, and clinicians and researchers know much less about their likely cause and optimal treatment. Therefore, *DSM-5* simply provides brief descriptions (rather than detailed diagnostic criteria) so that clinicians can easily recognize them despite their unofficial status (see appendix A). The five subtypes include

1. *Atypical anorexia nervosa* (anorexic features without low weight)

2. *Subthreshold** *bulimia nervosa* (bingeing and purging less than once per week)

---

* The terms "subthreshold" and "subclinical" can be used interchangeably to describe psychiatric diagnoses.

3. *Subthreshold binge eating disorder* (binge eating less than once per week)

4. *Purging disorder* (purging without binge eating)

5. *Night eating syndrome* (a pattern of eating very late in the evening, or in the middle of the night)

Emma's doctor, noting that her weight was not significantly low despite her dangerous loss of pounds, would specifically diagnose her with atypical anorexia nervosa. During her recovery journey, Jenni would have fallen at different points along the anorexic continuum, including many of the OSFED variations.

People often feel invalidated by the OSFED diagnosis, sharing Emma's disappointment that they are not quite "sick enough" to have anorexia nervosa. In her outreach work, Jenni has connected with countless individuals who have had difficulty making sense of the acronym. For example, Elijah Corbin, who identifies as nongender identity, told her, "Whereas mental health professionals have often reacted with confusion to explanations of my nongender identity, it is myself who has reacted with confusion to being in treatment for an eating disorder. I've seen too many mental health professionals to be convinced of diagnostic consistency, so the idea of OSFED only tugs at my general skepticism. I go through bouts of complete doubt that I have an eating disorder at all—I'm not anorexic, right? And I'm not bulimic, right? So how could I have an eating disorder?"[2] Similarly, journalist Carrie Arnold used the diagnostic criteria to deny that she had a problem. As she describes in her first-hand recovery account *Next to Nothing*, "My eating disorder told me I wasn't thin enough to

45

have anorexia. Ed said that if there was anyone in the world who was thinner than I, I couldn't be anorexic. My periods hadn't stopped. I binged and purged occasionally, but not enough to meet the criteria for bulimia. Even when I was desperately ill and in the emergency room for the third time in a week, I still didn't believe I had an eating disorder."[3] Similarly, Constance Rhodes, author of *Life Inside the "Thin" Cage*, used her subclinical eating diagnosis as a reason to avoid getting help. "I don't have an eating disorder. I just watch what I eat," she told concerned friends and family.[4]

When they were struggling, what Emma, Elijah, Carrie, and Constance did not realize is that subclinical eating disorders are often just as devastating as the officially recognized illnesses. To test this hypothesis, Dr. Thomas carried out a meta-analysis of 125 studies from 1987 to 2007 that compared individuals with subclinical eating disorders to those who met full criteria for anorexia, bulimia nervosa, and binge eating disorder.[5] (A meta-analysis is a powerful study design in which researchers statistically average findings across many different studies, in order to draw stronger conclusions than they can from a single investigation.) Dr. Thomas's work revealed that, averaging across studies, those with subclinical eating disorders scored just as high on degree of eating pathology (e.g., drive for thinness and body image disturbance) and general psychopathology (e.g., depression and anxiety) as those with anorexia and binge eating disorder, and just as low on measures of physical health (e.g., reduced bone density and gastrointestinal disorders) as those with anorexia. When it came to bulimia, individuals with subclinical eating disorders actually had more severe physical health problems, and they scored only slightly lower on eating pathology and general psychopathology. Subclinical eating disorders can even predict the onset of a diverse array of future mental health problems. In a recent longitudinal study, young girls with subclinical eating disorders were significantly more likely than their peers without eating disorders to develop depressive symptoms, begin binge drinking frequently, and start using street drugs as they entered adolescence and young adulthood.[6]

In summary, almost anorexia can be on the same level—just as serious—as officially recognized *DSM-5* eating disorders. Its position in the gray zone of the anorexic continuum is merely a consequence of constantly evolving diagnostic criteria, which represent clinical researchers' best guess at defining anorexia but are admittedly somewhat arbitrary. Even at the residential eating disorder treatment program where Dr. Thomas has conducted her research, approximately one-third of patients do not meet criteria for anorexia, bulimia, or binge eating disorder and can only be diagnosed with OSFED.[7] If you see yourself in any of the five subtype descriptions or if you feel that eating and weight control your life, please know that you do not have to continue living this way. Don't use diagnostic criteria as a way to talk yourself out of taking steps toward positive change.

Almost Anorexic Today, Anorexic Tomorrow

Another reason it is important to take almost anorexia seriously is that many individuals with almost anorexia will eventually develop anorexia nervosa. When Jenni's weight plummeted during her first semester in college, she had already begun this insidious progression. Without help, her illness was becoming more severe in terms of weight loss, putting her at increasingly greater risk for physical health problems.

In his book *Just a Little Too Thin*,[8] clinical psychologist Michael Strober described the development of anorexia in three phases, starting with "innocent dieting," progressing to "exhilarated dieting," and culminating in the "obsessed and preoccupied dieting" that is characteristic of full-blown anorexia nervosa. Similarly, researchers at the University of Sydney have suggested that anorexia should be labeled in stages, much like cancer (which is categorized from stage 1 to stage 4), so that milder and short-lived forms of the illness can be identified and treated before they become the opposite: severe and chronic.[9] For example, if Jenni had been diagnosed with "stage 1 anorexia" prior to entering college, perhaps she never would have progressed to "stage 4," where she ultimately developed hypotension (low blood pressure), bradycardia (low heart rate), and osteoporosis. Also significant to point out is that consequences of her almost anorexia—hair loss, poor concentration, and feeling cold all the time—only became worse as her illness progressed. Without question, studies indicate that treating anorexia in its early phases—that is, catching almost anorexia before it becomes full-blown anorexia—is much more effective than waiting until things get worse. And, without treatment, they usually do.

Based on this information, in part, the official criteria for anorexia have become broader over the past four decades. Earlier versions of *DSM* required a weight loss of at least 25 percent of an individual's original body weight to make a diagnosis of anorexia nervosa; later versions suggested that individuals should weigh just 15 percent below their expected weight (that is, the national average for age and height). Most recently, the new *DSM* has omitted the weight requirement entirely to encourage clinicians to use their own judgment to decide whether a patient's weight is significantly low. Similarly, whereas amenorrhea (the loss of menstrual periods for at least three months) was required in earlier versions, *DSM-5* has dropped this measure as well, in part because it cannot be applied to men or young people. This means that not long ago, many people whom we view as clearly having anorexia today wouldn't have received the diagnosis—based solely on some words that changed in a book.

Interestingly enough, the progression from almost anorexia to anorexia due to weight loss seemingly helps some people feel better about their bodies—because they are thinner. In one study, those with almost anorexia who were at a normal or above-average weight reported significantly worse body image than those with anorexia nervosa.[10] In other words, one person's pain cannot be compared to another's simply by looking at which *DSM* category he or she happens to fall into on a given day.

Anorexic Today, Almost Anorexic Tomorrow

No, this subheading is not a mistake. Almost anorexia can be not only a precursor to a full-fledged eating disorder but, as it was for Jenni, also a phase that many people pass through on their way to full recovery. Writer Marya Hornbacher captured this phase well in her anorexia memoir *Wasted:* "This is the very boring part of eating disorders, the aftermath. When you eat and you hate that you eat . . . This state, when it is effectively Over, is haunting in its own way. . . . You do not qualify as an eating-disordered person. And you feel bad about this. You feel as if you really ought to count, you ought to still merit worry."[11]

Some individuals assume that after experiencing the ravages of anorexia nervosa, almost anorexia might be as good as it gets. A recent study interviewed women who had previously received eating disorder treatment and divided them into two groups. The first group had achieved normal weight, no longer engaged in bingeing or purging, and scored similarly to healthy individuals on a standard measure of disordered-eating attitudes. The second group had also achieved normal weight and abstinence from bingeing and purging, but still experienced disordered attitudes. Interestingly, a similar proportion of each group identified themselves as "recovered."[12]

Aimee Liu, who herself recovered from anorexia nervosa, chronicled the recovery paths of women with eating disorders in her book *Gaining*. She noted that many of them had made great progress in stopping destructive food behaviors but still battled a persistent eating-disorder mind-set. For instance, "Sally," a pseudonym Liu used to describe one of her interviewees, suffered with bulimia from ages fifteen to twenty-two. Although she had finally stopped vomiting, Sally "still had a very bulimic way of seeing the world." According to Liu, Sally "binged and purged" on "kickboxing, marathon running, rollerblading, spinning, Pilates, foreign vacations, home decorating and entertaining, as well as professional megaprojects, and, on occasion, friends."[13] At one time or another, most people with disordered eating end up in this phase. And that last word—

phase—is very important. Don't get stuck in a place that is meant for moving through. All too often, almost anorexia is a way station between full-blown eating disorder and full-blown recovery.

Jenni's Journey

Ed never liked the idea of recovery. If I got better, he was out of a job. In the beginning, he wasn't too worried about my efforts, thinking that I would never succeed. But when he started to see that I had made some progress, he changed his tactic: *If I can't have all of Jenni, I must keep at least part of her—forever.* This is when Ed started acting like he supported my recovery. He would say things like, "Sure, Jenni, eat all of your meals today— just don't ever eat any high-fat foods." But this kind of behavior—holding on to any part of Ed—would eventually lead me back to him full force. I think Ed knew that too. When I inevitably fell headfirst into his arms again, I would grumble, "It's not my fault. Ed has me in a death grip and won't let go." Ed surely was holding on tight, but that didn't matter. Maybe I couldn't peel Ed off of me, but I could take accountability for my own actions. The point of separating from Ed, of seeing my eating disorder as separate from myself, was to put me in a position to say no to him and yes to life. If I decided to agree with him instead, I made that choice—I couldn't blame Ed for it. Make no mistake: I never chose to have an eating disorder, but I did choose recovery. And, ultimately, I resolved to reach a full recovery—pushing past the almost anorexic phase. Sometimes, I had to choose recovery one day at a time, one meal at a time, and even one moment at a time. Is there anything that you need to do in this very moment? Be careful, Ed is probably chiming in with ideas right now. Find your voice instead, and choose life.

Jeans or Genes?

Although we do not know exactly what causes almost anorexia and other officially recognized eating disorders, we know a great deal more now than we used to. Experts once hotly debated the role of jeans—environment—versus genes—familial inheritance—but now the field accepts that each plays a vital and synergistic role.

Jeans

With countless men and women currently dieting to fit into their "skinny jeans," it's no secret that cultural pressures for thinness contribute to eating disorder risk. In a fascinating natural experiment conducted when television was introduced to the island nation of Fiji, psychiatrist and social anthropologist Anne Becker observed a dramatic increase in the prevalence of almost anorexia. When Dr. Becker interviewed a group of media-naive adolescent girls just a few weeks after television arrived, none of them reported vomiting to control their weight, and only 13 percent scored above the clinical cutoff on a standard measure of eating disorder symptoms. But when she returned to Fiji three years later to interview a new crop of teen girls who had been exposed to American television shows (think *Melrose Place* and *Beverly Hills 90210*) during their formative years, 11 percent were vomiting, and 30 percent scored above the clinical cutoff for eating disorder symptoms.[14] These data provide a powerful illustration of how the propagation of the thin ideal can promote disordered eating. Environmental influences may not only affect whether someone develops an eating disorder but may also shape the specific symptoms a person develops. For example, in culturally non-Western societies that place less emphasis on the thin ideal, a common form of almost anorexia comprises all the recognizable features of anorexia nervosa—except the intense fear of weight gain.[15]

Genes

Given that cultural pressures for thinness are ubiquitous, whereas almost anorexia is not, it logically follows that some individuals are more vulnerable to developing disordered eating than others. Indeed, research suggests that disordered eating runs in families. For example, the parents, children, and siblings of individuals with anorexia nervosa are eleven times more likely to have anorexia themselves and six times more likely to have almost anorexia, compared to relatives of individuals without eating disorders.[16] This could be due in part to role modeling of disordered eating from one family member to another. Dr. Thomas recently evaluated an eleven-year-old girl for anorexia, while the girl's concerned mother (who was also underweight) sat in the waiting room reading a popular diet book. However, such cases are the exception rather than the rule, and adoption and twin studies suggest that genes play a much more important role than family environment in promoting eating disorder risk. For example, adopted children's eating disorder symptoms resemble those of their biological siblings—not their adoptive ones.[17] Similarly, if one member of a twin pair has anorexia nervosa or almost anorexia, the likelihood of his or her twin having either disorder is much greater if the twins are identical (that is, sharing 100 percent of their genes) versus fraternal (that is, sharing just 50 percent of their genes, on average).[18] Taken together, family-based studies suggest that 50 to 80 percent of eating disorder risk is due to genetic effects. Importantly, these figures are very similar to those of other psychiatric disorders that we typically view as "biological," like schizophrenia and bipolar disorder. Not only do eating disorders themselves run in families, but the individual symptoms that comprise each *DSM-5* diagnosis—from drive for thinness to binge eating—are also partly genetic. This helps explain why there are so many different variations and subtypes of almost anorexia: You may have inherited risk for certain symptoms (such as body dissatisfaction) but not others (for example, purging). In summary, it's likely that "genes load the gun, but the environment pulls the trigger."[19]

Neurobiology

Psychiatrist Thomas Insel, director of the U.S. National Institute of Mental Health, has said, "Eating disorders are presumably brain disorders."[20] Some people and organizations have found brain-disorder language extremely helpful in explaining to others why individuals with eating disorders can't just "snap out of it" and in absolving parents of guilt and blame for their child's illness. Others, however, have worried that brain-disorder language may give sufferers and loved ones alike the hopeless (and false!) impression that eating disorders are lifelong illnesses that cannot be treated and may even provide a handy excuse for the continuation of dangerous symptoms (after all, your brain made you do it). To combat this, parent activist Laura Collins Lyster-Mensh has used the term "treatable brain disorder."[21] We suggest you use the terminology that works best for you. Words are powerful. Don't let Ed hijack them.

So, if eating disorders are in part genetic, what gets inherited, exactly? Researchers have yet to confirm the specific genes that confer risk, but distinctive personality traits and thinking styles are possible candidates. Individuals with eating disorders are typically perfectionistic, obsessive-compulsive, and sensitive to emotional pain. Clinical psychologist Lisa Lilenfeld, whose research focuses on personality traits associated with eating disorders, told us, "It is really unprecedented in any other area of psychopathology to see the homogeneity of personality presentation that we see in restricting-type anorexia nervosa."[22] Indeed, those with anorexia are typically anxious, detail oriented, and rule driven. In contrast, those with bulimia are often impulsive and risk taking.[23] Those who have symptoms of anorexia and bulimia, like Jenni did, typically have traits in both categories.

Neurobiological research indicates that people with eating disorders exhibit brain abnormalities that may at least partially explain symptoms. According to psychiatrist Walter Kaye, "Studies suggest those with anorexia nervosa have increased activity of the brain's serotonin system, which could play a role in high anxiety. Since serotonin is made from an essential amino acid that can only be obtained from the diet, it is possible that restricting food intake is a means of reducing serotonin and thus feeling less anxious."[24] The strong preference for rigid rules and routines among individuals with anorexia may also be encoded in neural circuits. In one study, subjects were placed in a brain scanner while performing a task in which they were asked to identify whether each new shape that flashed on the screen in front of them was the same or different from a reference shape (either a triangle or a circle) that frequently changed. Compared to healthy controls, those with anorexia made more errors when the reference shape changed. In other words, when they had to update their routine (that is, begin comparing the shape on the screen to a circle rather than a triangle or vice versa), they made more errors. They also exhibited lower activation in the frontal-striatal-thalamic loop, a brain network associated with cognitive flexibility, while performing this task.[25]

Repurposing Positive Eating Disorder Traits

Maintaining disordered eating is pretty challenging, and in many ways it requires a great deal of skill. Someone who restricts food, for example, has the ability to delay gratification, a trait that can be very helpful if you are trying to complete a work project or wait for late party guests to arrive. In one study, anorexia patients were willing to wait significantly longer to receive a hypothetical amount of money compared to healthy controls.[26] Have you used some of your best personality traits in the service of disordered eating? See table 2 which follows for a list of positive traits commonly associated with almost anorexia and other officially recognized eating disorders.[27] You might be thinking that some of the examples don't look very positive, but all of the traits listed, in fact, can be. For example, perfectionism might be viewed as the pursuit of excellence and obsessive-compulsiveness as conscientiousness. If you see yourself in any of these traits, rest assured that you can harness the good in all of them. Follow Jenni's example from table 2, and take some time to think about your traits. Then place marks in table 3 next to the ones that you notice in your life, or write down those traits in a notebook.

Now make a list of large or small goals. These might be related to recovery, life in general, or both. Similar to Jenni's example, match traits that might help you to achieve each goal.

BECOMING ALMOST ANOREXIC ❖

Table 2.

Matching Jenni's Positive Traits to Life Goals

This table shows Jenni's responses in early Ed recovery.

Positive traits commonly associated with almost anorexia and other officially recognized eating disorders		
General Eating Disorder Traits	**Anorexic Traits**	**Bulimic Traits**
Perfectionism √	Persistence √	Impulsivity —
Obsessive-compulsiveness √	Low risk-taking —	Risk-taking —
Sensitivity to emotional pain √	Attention to detail √	Need for new experiences √
Intelligence √	Preference for routine √	Intolerance of routine —
	Ability to delay gratification √	

Jenni's goals for the next 6 months	**Traits that will help her pursue these goals**
1. Don't skip meals (even if I feel guilty)	1. Ability to delay gratification, perfectionism
2. Go to Monday night group therapy	2. Persistence, preference for routine
3. Do something fun with friends weekly	3. Persistence, perfectionism, attention to detail
4. Write a new song	4. Sensitivity to emotional pain, need for new experiences
5. Perform songs at a local café	5. Obsessive-compulsiveness, attention to detail, intelligence

Table 3.

Matching Your Positive Traits to Life Goals

Positive traits commonly associated with almost anorexia and other officially recognized eating disorders		
General Eating Disorder Traits	Anorexic Traits	Bulimic Traits
Perfectionism ___	Persistence ___	Impulsivity ___
Obsessive-compulsiveness ___	Low risk-taking ___	Risk-taking ___
Sensitivity to emotional pain ___	Attention to detail ___	Need for new experiences ___
Intelligence ___	Preference for routine ___	Intolerance of routine ___
	Ability to delay gratification ___	

My goals for the next 6 months	Traits that will help me pursue these goals
1.	1.
2.	2.
3.	3.
4.	4.
5.	5.

This table can be downloaded at www.almostanorexic.com.

You already have the qualities you need to move forward in your life. It's just a matter of repurposing your valuable traits in the service of health and happiness instead of illness.

Is Everyone Almost Anorexic?

Some would answer yes to the question this subheading poses. Clinical psychologist Stacey Rosenfeld frequently writes about her belief that "every woman has an eating disorder" in her blog of the same name. She has written, "My contention is that every woman has an eating disorder—not necessarily anorexia or bulimia per se, but a fixation on food/weight/shape that is unhealthy, unwanted, and undying."[28] While we don't believe that every woman (or man, for that matter) has an eating disorder, we definitely understand where she is coming from.

After repeatedly being told by people who had read her books, "I don't have an eating disorder, but I do have an Ed in my head," Jenni decided to name the voice that seemingly everyone was hearing. It was almost like society itself had an eating disorder, so, in her second book, *Goodbye Ed, Hello Me*, she named that voice "Societal Ed." Do you hear Societal Ed? Unless you are living on a deserted island without wi-fi or cell service, then you probably do. Societal Ed lives in so many places—from movies and television to magazines and online advertisements—that you can hardly avoid hearing "his" pervasive message that our bodies aren't good enough. Even Dr. Thomas, whose career is devoted to helping people feel better about their bodies, knows the singular frustration of a bad hair day. We all might hear Societal Ed, but we don't all have eating disorders. And we definitely don't all have to listen.

If you are almost anorexic, Societal Ed might speak louder and more frequently to you than to someone who doesn't struggle. But the good news is that you, too, can learn to stop listening. If distinguishing between your personal Ed and Societal Ed is confusing to you, then don't worry about the difference at this point. Further down the recovery road, this distinction will become important. When you are fully recovered (and you can be), you still might hear a voice from time to time that says to "eat less" and "lose a few pounds." This is when it becomes essential to understand that the voice you are hearing is not your personal Ed rearing its ugly head again but rather the one that we all hear—Societal Ed. Yes, you can kick Ed out of your life for good.

Prevalence of Almost Anorexia

Although it is impossible to determine exactly how many people are struggling, available data suggest that almost anorexia is significantly more common than anorexia itself. Because epidemiological studies are designed to assess the prevalence of many psychiatric problems across thousands of people, they typically include just a few questions about eating disorders. So researchers must carefully choose the questions most likely to identify individuals with officially recognized eating disorders and cannot typically capture all possible forms of almost anorexia. This means that the true number of people who have almost anorexia is probably underestimated by population-based studies.

With this in mind, the best prevalence estimates come from the National Comorbidity Survey Replication, which assessed several, though not all, forms of EDNOS (here's that long acronym again—eating disorders not otherwise specified) in a nationally representative sample of adults eighteen and older. Nearly eight times as many people reported a lifetime history of a subclinical eating disorder (4.6 percent) compared to those who reported anorexia nervosa (0.6 percent).[29] In other words, for every adult who has experienced full syndrome anorexia (roughly 1 in 200), many more (at least 1 in 20) have struggled with almost anorexia. And available data suggest that almost anorexia is even more prevalent among adolescent females, the demographic group at highest risk for eating disorders, with a prevalence ranging from 12 percent (just over 1 in 10) to 15 percent (3 in 20).[30]

The Difference between Almost Anorexia and Normal Eating

If only 1 in 20 adults have almost anorexia, it naturally follows that 19 in 20 do not. Dieting to fit into a prom dress or wedding tux doesn't make you almost anorexic, nor does trying to eat fewer desserts for a couple of weeks or running a five-kilometer charity race with your friends. With the majority of American adults classified as overweight, it is no surprise that many are trying to eat more nutritiously. And of course, moderate exercise can be healthy and fun—just ask Jenni; she has two mountain bikes.

However, each of these examples could lead to almost anorexia if they become rigid patterns of behavior. If you are dieting to fit into every article of clothing in your closet, if you never allow yourself to eat sweets even though you love chocolate, or if you force yourself to run on the treadmill every morning despite being injured or sick, these could be important red flags. Counterintuitively, the very thing you might expect to be the biggest red flag for almost anorexia actually isn't the best indicator—the number on the scale.

3

Underweight, Overweight, and Everything in Between

Do you step on a bathroom scale every morning to check your weight? For some, this single number provides a ready answer to a host of questions—from the mundane to the existential. *Can I still fit into my favorite jeans? Is today going to be a good day? Am I worthy of love?* Unfortunately, many people with almost anorexia also let the scale tell them whether they should seek help. They may mistakenly believe that they are not sick enough —or rather, thin enough—to have a real problem with food. But you don't have to be super-skinny to have almost anorexia. People of all shapes and sizes struggle with disordered-eating attitudes and behaviors.

Don't Call Me Anorexic

Celebrity tabloids may hand out just as many anorexia diagnoses per year as qualified health care professionals. Nearly every week, the cover of *Star, In Touch,* or *OK!* identifies yet another ultrathin celebrity, politician, or royal family member whom they think must have an eating disorder. Allegations typically persist even when public figures deny them, creating controversy and boosting magazine sales in the process.

Disordered eating exists at every number on the scale. This means that being underweight does not automatically rule a person into the anorexic or almost anorexic category. Although we can't say for sure whether any given celebrity has an eating disorder, we do know that anorexia is just one possible reason for a low body weight. People can be underweight because they smoke, are physically ill, are under stress, or are simply small because of their body type and genes.[1]

Likewise, a healthy, normal-weight appearance does not make someone immune to disordered eating. The petite but curvy Demi Lovato shocked music fans when she admitted herself to a residential eating disorder treatment facility for bulimia in 2010. In her documentary *Stay Strong*, the singer publicly described her long-standing struggle with restricting and self-induced vomiting. She remembered that, before seeking treatment, "I knew that I'd lost weight, I knew that what I was doing was wrong, but I never could admit that I had a problem because I never thought that it was bad enough. You know, I always thought, I don't have a problem because I'm not X amount of pounds."[2]

Dr. Thomas's own patients frequently tell her that they are "too fat" to have an eating disorder, despite their dangerous restricting, bingeing, or purging behaviors. Some have admitted to cutting calories in the weeks prior to beginning therapy because they were worried that they wouldn't qualify for treatment at their current weight. She often spends a good portion of her first session with new patients simply explaining that, if they felt concerned enough to make an appointment, they have every right to be sitting in her office.

Not Just a Number

Many people struggling with almost anorexia feel compelled to reach a specific target weight in order to legitimize their problems with food. Previous versions of the diagnostic criteria have provided specific guidelines for the weight at which anorexia nervosa might be diagnosed. *DSM-IV,* for instance, included an example of less than 85 percent of expected weight. "Unfortunately, that example was often interpreted as a strict limit, which was not the intent," psychiatrist Tim Walsh told us.[3] He chaired both the *DSM-IV* and *DSM-5* Eating Disorder Work Groups that created the diagnostic criteria.

Early career lawyer Adam Lamparello certainly interpreted it that way. In his eating disorder recovery memoir, *Ten-Mile Morning,* Adam recalled working out for six hours per day and restricting his diet primarily to raw vegetables, yet still feeling ashamed that his weight fell above "the 'golden' weight that defines you as officially anorexic." He knew that "I would earn the 'anorexia' label if my weight fell fifteen percent below the normal range for my size." At the height of his illness, reaching this arbitrary target became "my most important goal up to this point in my life."[4]

Although a number like 85 percent might sound pretty precise (after all, it's math!), there is actually a great deal of variation in how medical professionals define the boundary between low and normal weight. Dr. Thomas, for example, works at two Harvard-affiliated eating disorder programs that use totally different methods of calculating expected weight. Although each one is perfectly reasonable and supported by science, they nonetheless produce different anorexia cutoff points for the exact same patients. One of Dr. Thomas's recent patients, who sought help from professionals at both programs, was diagnosed with anorexia at one and almost anorexia at the other—and on the same day!

Indeed, literally dozens of methods can be used to calculate expected weight for height, and each one results in a different cutoff for the "anorexic" range. Dr. Thomas's review of 99 anorexia studies identified ten different methods for calculating a person's expected weight—ranging from specific BMI values to various normative weight tables. (Remember that BMI stands for body mass index.) Comparing the lowest expected weights to the highest revealed large discrepancies in the body size at which anorexia would be diagnosed. The difference between the strictest and most lenient cutoff point was fifteen pounds for females and twenty-six pounds for males.[5] Ironically, Adam probably could have reached his life's goal by simply using a different weight chart.

Fortunately, researchers and clinicians are taking steps to ensure that individuals with eating disorders don't use the number on the scale to sidestep seeking help. According to Dr. Walsh, "In order to avoid this problem, in *DSM-5*, the Work Group decided it would be best to include no numerical guideline regarding weight in the criteria."[6] Instead, the text includes guidance for determining how underweight each patient is on a case-by-case basis.

But You Don't Look Like You Have an Eating Disorder

Tragically, people can die from eating disorders even if they "look normal." At only nineteen years old, Andrea Smeltzer was one.

Throughout her thirteen-month struggle with restricting, binge eating, and purging, Andrea's weight always fell within the normal range. Her mother, Doris Smeltzer, who commemorated her daughter's life in a memoir called *Andrea's Voice*,[7] told us, "On the day that Andrea died, she was the picture of health." Just hours before her death, Andrea had gone on her nightly walk, which was, according to Doris, "a ridiculous number of miles." Doris said, "I imagine those who saw her pass by their homes in the quaint village of Claremont, California, may have silently given her an 'at-a-girl' for 'taking such good care of herself.'"[8]

But the health consequences of purging are insidious, and what no one realized was that, despite Andrea's healthy appearance, her potassium was getting dangerously low. (Frequent vomiting depletes the body of important salts—such as potassium, sodium, and chloride—that are necessary for maintaining the electrical impulses that help our muscles contract.) That night, Andrea died in her sleep from an electrolyte imbalance that caused her heart (one of the body's most important muscles) to stop.

Like the officially recognized eating disorders anorexia, bulimia, and binge eating disorder, almost anorexia can be deadly. Unfortunately, accurate mortality statistics can be difficult to pin down, as the majority of death certificates don't cite the eating disorder as the immediate cause of death. Andrea's, for example, cites "undetermined." Others list cardiac arrest or suicide. However, a recent study used the National Death Index to retrospectively track all-cause mortality among patients at a large outpatient eating disorder clinic. ("All-cause" refers to death from any cause, whether related to an eating disorder or not.) Even though patients with anorexia were underweight, whereas those with bulimia and EDNOS were normal weight,

Jenni's Journey

I was thin. I wasn't. My size fluctuated throughout my struggle with disordered eating and well into my recovery. I sometimes looked different, but the pain on the inside was always the same. From friends to even some health care professionals, people just didn't seem to understand that. "You don't look like you have an eating disorder," a doctor once said to me. With this one ignorant comment, I felt unworthy and out of place. *Do I need to lose more weight in order to get help?* Later on, when I had found another doctor to help me and had finally gained some much-needed weight in recovery, friends said excitedly, "You look so healthy. I'm glad you're better." Again, I felt puzzled and misunderstood. *Why do people keep using my body as the barometer for how I am doing in life and recovery?* I wasn't better. At that point, I had stopped compensating for binges (but was bingeing more than ever), so I had actually gained weight fast. While learning to not compensate for a binge was, in fact, a positive turning point in my recovery, it was difficult for me to believe that since Ed was constantly yelling, "You are a failure." I felt worse. If your loved one struggles, remember to ask how he or she is doing on the inside. You can't tell just by looking. If you have almost anorexia, you might need to teach people, like I did: There is no certain way an eating disorder—or recovery—looks. Anyone of any size might suffer. But, more importantly, with support, anyone can get better too.

mortality was similar across groups. Over the eight- to twenty-five-year follow-up period, 5.2 percent of EDNOS patients died, compared to 4.0 percent of those with anorexia and 3.9 percent of individuals with bulimia.[9]

The take-home message? Disordered eating can have serious health consequences—at whatever number on the scale.

I Don't Have an Eating Disorder—I Eat Too Much

People tend to minimize not only the legitimacy of eating problems at normal weight but also the validity of disorders involving overeating. Dr. Thomas recently went to an academic conference attended by a diverse range of mental health professionals. When she explained to a fellow psychologist that she was conducting a study on binge eating disorder, he chuckled and joked, "Oh, I binge all the time! If there were a bowl of M&M's in front of me right now, I would eat the whole thing." But disorders involving loss of control over eating at normal or even higher weights—such as binge eating disorder, bulimia nervosa, and some forms of almost anorexia—are no laughing matter.

Scientific studies suggest that, unlike anorexic behaviors, bulimic and binge-eating behaviors do not lie on a continuum with normal eating.[10] In other words, although the vast majority of young women have gone on a diet,[11] true bingeing (that is, eating large amounts of food while feeling out of control) and purging (that is, trying to compensate for overeating through vomiting, laxatives, or diuretics) differ categorically from normal eating. This is yet another reason why we named this book *Almost Anorexic* rather than *Almost Bulimic* or *Almost Binge Eating Disorder.*

Bulimia Nervosa

Bulimia nervosa involves recurrent binge eating followed by compensatory behaviors (such as self-induced vomiting, laxative use, or fasting) that are designed to "make up for" the calories consumed. People often binge despite not feeling particularly hungry. They may eat quickly and secretively so as to avoid being discovered. They often don't stop until they feel uncomfortably full and very guilty. What Dr. Thomas's colleague did not understand was that just eating a few extra M&M's isn't a binge. Most people eat more M&M's (or any tasty food) out of a large bowl than a single-serving pack. True bingeing, on the other hand, involves an extremely large quantity of food and the desperate feeling that you *can't stop* eating.

The *DSM-5* criteria (see appendix A) require that you binge and purge at least once a week for three months to receive a diagnosis of bulimia. Does that mean that bingeing and purging once a month is healthy? Of course not. Even people who binge and purge infrequently share a dangerous mind-set that overemphasizes the importance of being thin.[12] In other words, when it comes to food and weight, Ed still calls the shots. That's why subthreshold bulimia nervosa—a pattern of occasional bingeing and compensatory behaviors—is another form of almost anorexia.

It is important to note that those who binge and purge while clinically underweight are diagnosed with anorexia nervosa (binge/purge type). People with bulimia and subthreshold bulimia are typically normal weight and, increasingly in clinical settings, overweight.[13] This is yet another reason to disregard the number on the scale when it comes to seeking help.

Binge Eating Disorder

Prior to the publication of *DSM-5*, binge eating disorder, commonly called BED, was not listed as an officially recognized eating disorder in this diagnostic manual. It hid in the appendix of the book, because researchers didn't know enough about its causes and treatment. Referring to the official recognition of BED, Chevese Turner, who founded the Binge Eating Disorder Association and herself struggled with the illness, told us, "It is essential that we now begin, in earnest, to educate the general public that eating disorders affect people of every size."[14]

Just like bulimia, binge eating disorder involves recurrent bingeing. However, unlike bulimia, people with binge eating disorder do not use compensatory behaviors (see appendix A). This doesn't mean that people with binge eating disorder don't care about their weight. Most of them do. Many of Dr. Thomas's patients with binge eating disorder are overweight or obese, and they have struggled with chronic dieting their entire lives. In a recent study, more than two-thirds of adults with binge eating disorder reported that changes in shape and weight were among the most important determinants of their self-esteem.[15] Ironically, it is often this weight-loss mind-set that fuels binge eating. This is why subthreshold binge eating disorder, a pattern of occasional binge eating accompanied by marked distress, is another form of almost anorexia.

Not all overweight people who struggle with disordered eating have binge eating disorder. And, contrary to what many think, not all people with binge eating disorder are larger. Similar to bulimia, some are at a normal weight.

· · ·

As we said before, an individual who meets some but not all of the criteria for bulimia nervosa or binge eating disorder would fall into the almost anorexic category. Abriana, who struggles with subthreshold binge eating disorder, is one.

Abriana

Abriana's favorite poem was "Desiderata" by Max Erhmann. She especially loved the line, "You are a child of the universe, no less than the trees and the stars; you have a right to be here," mainly because she desperately wanted to believe it.

She first realized she was overweight at age eleven. She had spent the especially hot summer afternoon at her friend Tanya's house, running in the sprinklers. As the scent of freshly baked cookies wafted into the backyard, the two girls grinned at each other and raced to the kitchen, where Tanya's mom was carefully sliding the chocolate-studded morsels out of the oven. "Here, teeny Tanya, you can have two," her mother smiled. Then, poking Abriana's stomach disapprovingly, Tanya's mother asked, "Why don't you start with just one?"

Abriana felt like she'd been slapped. She declined the cookie in shame. *I am such a fat, disgusting pig,* she thought. *I don't deserve this treat.* Scrutinizing her bikini-clad body in her bathroom mirror that night, she wondered desperately why she didn't look more like pre-pubertal Tanya, with her flat stomach and skinny legs. Sucking in her stomach and squeezing the flesh of her thighs out of view, Abriana pinched herself so hard that she left angry red marks on her body.

From that day forward, she divided activities into two types: those for the Tanyas of the world, and those for the Abrianas. Not wanting to offend others with her oversized presence,

Abriana chose academics over sports, sweatshirts over tank tops, and television over parties. She threw herself into her studies, thinking, *At least fat girls can still get into Ivy League schools.* During her first semester in college, Abriana unintentionally won the affection of a young man named Daniel. When he first asked her out, she was beside herself. *Why would anyone want to date me?* She said yes reluctantly, but after their first date at the school's dining hall, they both had a feeling that they were meant to be. Daniel never understood why she hated her body so much and hoped that his marriage proposal would change her mind about how she looked.

Despite Daniel's insistence throughout their thirty-year marriage that he thought she was beautiful, Abriana tried everything to lose weight. She was a self-proclaimed "chronic dieter," but she didn't necessarily believe it was a problem. (It was.) Spending countless dollars on over-the-counter diet pills, meal replacement bars, and weight-loss club memberships, she also amassed an impressive collection of workout DVDs based on every conceivable fitness theory—from aerobic intervals to muscle confusion. She even made her cell phone ring tone the sound of an oinking pig, to remind her not to snack between her meager mini-meals. But nothing ever worked. The heady optimism of each new weight-loss program was always punctuated by a bout of overeating and self-loathing. As soon as she ate one morsel of food outside the diet plan, she thought that she'd blown it. Every month or two, she would drive from one fast-food restaurant to another, eating a total of what might have been ten or more meals combined. *I have absolutely no self-control,* she thought. Inevitably, she felt disgusted with herself.

One place where Abriana could shed her mantle of self-doubt was at work. A charismatic litigator, she was proud of graduating from Columbia Law School and shattering the glass ceiling to become the first African American partner at a prestigious firm. Although she felt very much at home in the courtroom, the break room—which became a backdrop for her continued dieting efforts—was a different story. One day, while microwaving her low-calorie frozen meal to eat quickly before her lunchtime power walk, she saw a flyer advertising a firm-wide "biggest loser" competition, promising prizes and notoriety to the attorney who lost the most weight. As her colleagues began approaching her in the halls encouraging her to join up, she felt awash with shame. When one male partner pinched her stomach for emphasis, she bristled, immediately feeling as though she were once again the chubby little girl running through Tanya's sprinklers. *I don't deserve to be here*, she thought.

But, as a lawyer, Abriana knew her rights. After talking it over with Daniel, she went straight to the firm's employee assistance program (EAP) to report the harassment the next day. The EAP counselor agreed to reprimand the offending partner, who had previously drawn similar complaints. Abriana was surprised, however, when the counselor also legitimized her lifelong challenge with food. In the past, people had generally recommended some new diet or another, confirming Abriana's belief that only weight loss could bolster her flagging self-esteem. But this counselor truly listened and explained, "Abriana, I don't think the biggest loser competition is going to be healthy for you. Have you considered talking to a professional about your relationship with food and weight?" Feeling skeptical, Abriana reluctantly agreed to make an appointment with a social worker.

She was not used to having her eating problem taken seriously. After all, she was obese. But her new therapist explained, "Your ideal weight might never be what you want it to be. You may never be a size ten, but you can still be healthy. You can learn to see yourself how Daniel always has—as beautiful. And you can have peace with food." Abriana gained confidence as she began focusing less of her energy on dieting. And when the partner finally got fired after yet another harassment allegation from a female colleague, she thought to herself, *Maybe, just maybe, I do have a right to be here.*

A Dose of Reality

It may seem counterintuitive that heavier people can have almost anorexia, since a defining feature of anorexia nervosa is being underweight. But overweight individuals like Abriana are, in fact, at risk. In the past decade, a new crop of reality television shows has glorified restrictive diets and excessive exercise regimens—especially among those who are overweight. Most famously, on *The Biggest Loser*—the show that inspired the competition in Abriana's workplace—contestants vie for a monetary prize bestowed on the one who loses the most weight. Similarly, reality shows like *I Used to Be Fat* and *Too Fat for 15* promote the implicit message that less of someone is better—no matter what it takes to get there.

But former *Biggest Loser* finalist Kai Hibbard knows the truth. On television, season 3 viewers cheered Kai on as she lost 118 pounds, going from obese to a normal size in a matter of weeks. Her persistence in completing the *Biggest Loser* triathlon and riding a stationary bike suspended thirty feet in the air (despite her fear of heights) were an inspiration to rapt viewers at home. But what people did not see on camera were the dangerous techniques Kai was using to lose weight so quickly. She later revealed to reporters that, in addition to fasting, she put on multiple layers of clothes and worked out in 100-degree Fahrenheit temperatures.[16] Even though dehydrating herself was a dangerous behavior that only shed water—not fat—Kai became obsessed with decreasing the number on the scale at her weekly weigh-ins. According to Kai, while competing, she developed "an eating disorder that I battle every day."[17] As she told the *Early Show*, "I left with a very poor mental body image, I found myself loathing what I looked like the more weight I dropped because of the pressure on me. And I found myself doing things like considering coffee a meal. And because of the mentality that I was surrounded with, and the pressure that was given at that show, it was considered acceptable to behave that way."[18]

Reality shows like this dangerously, not to mention falsely, suggest that people who are larger do not have to worry about developing almost anorexia or other officially recognized eating disorders. And it is not just television spreading this message. Think about the extra-large "I beat anorexia" T-shirts that are marketed to obese individuals as novelty items. But research suggests that many people who struggle with almost anorexia are overweight, not emaciated. Dr. Thomas and her colleagues recently conducted a study at a weight-loss clinic to determine what proportion of patients would meet criteria for an eating disorder. Because this clinic's mission is to offer nutritional, psychological, and surgical support for individuals whose BMIs exceed 30, the findings might surprise you. In a structured clinical interview, more than one-third of these patients exhibited some form of disordered eating. Although a handful met *DSM-5* criteria for bulimia and binge eating disorder, the majority of those who struggled had some form of almost anorexia, including night eating syndrome, subthreshold binge eating disorder, subthreshold bulimia nervosa, purging disorder, or other subclinical eating problems.[19] In other words, the study showed that obesity does not protect people from developing almost anorexia and other officially recognized eating disorders. Indeed, it may put them at even greater risk.

Obese individuals seeking weight-loss surgery may be especially vulnerable. Studies suggest that about one-quarter of candidates evaluated for weight-loss surgery have binge eating disorder.[20] After undergoing surgery, many are able to stop bingeing, in part because their stomach capacity becomes so small. However, some postsurgical diet recommendations unwittingly mimic eating disorder behaviors (for example, patients are advised to eat very small portions, avoid high-sugar foods, and chew each bite meticulously to accommodate their now-smaller stomachs). Thus, a subset of patients is unable to shake the almost anorexic mind-set, even after they have achieved a healthy weight. Dr. Thomas has treated many individuals who have developed almost anorexia post-operatively, including some who began intentionally eating foods they knew would trigger "dumping syndrome" (a common surgical side effect that includes vomiting and diarrhea) so they could attempt to purge unwanted calories.

Can Dieting Make Me Fat?

Recent research sheds light on how disordered-eating behaviors like dieting can actually promote weight gain over time.

Diet ads commonly entice customers by comparing an over-weight "before" photo to a taut and toned "after" photo. But even if the after snapshot hasn't been airbrushed to perfection (which it probably has), this tactic is misleading. One study asked a large group of adolescent boys and girls over a ten-year period whether they engaged in behaviors such as fasting, eating very little food, using food substitutes (such as powders and special drinks), skipping meals, taking diet pills, self-inducing vomiting, or misusing laxatives/diuretics. Compared to their nondieting peers, adolescents who used dieting and unhealthy weight control behaviors gained significantly more weight over the course of the study.[21] Similarly, Dr. Thomas and her colleagues examined the relationship between breakfast skipping and body weight in a large sample of ethnic Fijian schoolgirls. Strikingly, 41 percent reported skipping breakfast at least three times per week, and frequent breakfast skipping was associated not only with disordered-eating attitudes, but also with higher odds of being overweight and obese.[22] No wonder diet ads don't show a third "after the after" photo—they probably wouldn't sell as many books, videos, and pills.

It may be tempting to assume that individuals who are genetically predisposed to higher weights are more likely to diet or skip meals in the first place. After all, they must want to lose weight. However, available data suggest that dieting itself may be the culprit. For example, identical twins share 100 percent of their genes but have different life experiences, making them an ideal population for disentangling genetic versus environmental effects. A recent study that tracked intentional weight-loss attempts and BMI over a nine-year period found that those who dieted actually gained more weight over time than their nondieting identical twins.[23] This may be because dieting creates chemical changes in our bodies that favor regaining any lost pounds. In one laboratory study, overweight and obese individuals who had lost an average of thirty pounds each over ten weeks had more of the appetite-promoting hormone ghrelin in their bloodstream one year later than they did before starting the weight-loss program.[24] No wonder they also reported feeling hungrier than they did the year before.

Taken together, these studies highlight the reciprocal relationship between dieting and weight gain, illustrating how almost anorexia—specifically chronic dieting—can be a cause of, rather than a cure for, obesity. Conversely, as we already described, being overweight and subsequently striving for weight loss can also lead to almost anorexia.

Almost Anorexia Is Not a Cure for Obesity

The current war on obesity leads people like Abriana to believe that eating less will make them healthier. The unintentional message seems to be that heavier individuals have a problem with food that can be solved simply by losing weight. Just think about the tagline of the recent HBO documentary series *The Weight of the Nation*: "To win, we have to lose." The focus is clearly on weight, not health. Dr. Thomas has worked with many overweight patients who have justified risky crash diets— subsisting for days on just juice or cabbage soup—as health-promoting escapes from obesity. In *Health at Every Size*, research psychologist Linda Bacon highlights the danger of this double standard: "Behaviors such as counting calories (or carbs or fat grams), using exercise to burn calories, [or] exercising several times a day . . . are suspicious when they come from an 'underweight' client, raising a red flag for eating disorders. But large clients who talk about these same behaviors are often applauded."[25]

Plain and simple, eating disorder symptoms are harmful regardless of body size. British television program *Supersize vs Superskinny*, however, portrays otherwise.[26] This popular reality show brings an obese person and an extremely underweight individual to live together for five days and asks them to swap diets. Sometimes, in a given day, the larger person is asked to drink copious cups of coffee and eat fewer than 1,000 calories, while the underweight individual is served junk foods and fast foods worth thousands of calories. The implication is that it is healthy for an obese individual to eat a severely restrictive diet and safe for someone with anorexia to regularly consume an extremely high-calorie diet, without any regard for the nutritional content. Both of these assumptions are dangerous.

While obesity is clearly associated with health problems and premature death, being overweight may not be the killer portrayed in the media. Many studies actually find a U-shaped association between BMI and mortality, with the longest life expectancy at a BMI of 25.[27] In one study, overweight Americans (that is, those with BMIs from 25.0 to 29.9) actually lived longer than those who were normal weight or obese.[28] That's why we recommend the same healthy behaviors—regular, nutritious meals and moderate exercise—to individuals of all shapes and sizes. If you are already obese, developing almost anorexia will just make matters worse.

Take Ragen Chastain, for example, the author of *Fat: The Owner's Manual*.[29] Ragen is obese by medical charts and, like many larger people, normal in terms of blood pressure, cholesterol, and other measures of physical health. A professional dancer, Ragen was once so concerned about her body that she restricted food to the point of developing an eating disorder. At her most ill, she was fueling her eight to ten hours of daily exercise with minimal calories, a dangerous practice that landed her in the hospital. Even then, she was not considered thin by societal standards. And she definitely wasn't healthy. After seeking professional treatment, Ragen ultimately regained her health and is currently, she says, "truly happy living completely outside the cultural beauty norm."[30]

Fat Is Not a Feeling (or Is It)?

Since almost anorexia can occur at any weight, it logically follows that people can "feel fat" at any shape. Indeed, one study of women (both with and without eating disorders) found no correlation between BMI and how "fat" participants felt; instead feelings of fatness were correlated with depression.[31] On the graph shown on the next page (figure 5) or in a notebook, rate the intensity of your feelings of fatness over the past week.

Typically, your weight stays relatively steady over the course of a week (or goes up or down by a small amount). However, feelings of fatness can fluctuate wildly. How can we account for this discrepancy? According to psychiatrist Christopher Fairburn, who developed this exercise as part of his innovative cognitive behavioral therapy for eating disorders, "Feeling fat is often the result of mislabeling of certain emotions and bodily experiences."[32] In other words, *I feel fat* is almost always code for something else: *I don't know what I'm feeling. I feel sad. I'm anxious.* When Ed told Jenni she was fat, she was often feeling lonely, angry, tired, or full. Usually, triggers other than changes

Figure 5.
Graph Your Feelings of Fatness for the Past Week
How fat have you felt in the past week?
Use this graph to rate the intensity of those feelings,
on a scale of 1 to 10, in the past seven days.

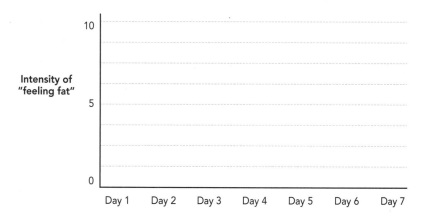

This exercise can be downloaded at www.almostanorexic.com.

in shape and weight influence how "fat" you feel at any given time. Abriana, for instance, was having fun playing in the sprinklers until Tanya's mom poked her stomach and told her to only have one cookie. Psychological triggers may include negative emotions such as shame, boredom, frustration, or irritability; eating (or just considering eating) a "fattening" food; or coming in contact with someone smaller than you. Jenni once wrote about feeling fat just because a thinner person stepped into an elevator next to her! In contrast, physiological triggers might include eating a filling meal, feeling physically ill, having your period, feeling overheated, or wearing tight-fitting clothing. The next time you are feeling fat, ask yourself, as Dr. Fairburn suggests: "What am I *really* feeling right now, and why?"[33]

Chances are good that you won't be able to change that feeling by simply going on a diet. Life is a lot more complicated than that.

4

Calories, Cleansing, and Colonics, Oh My!
Your Relationship with Food

When we came into this world, food was just food. None of us, as babies, wondered how many calories were in that jar of pureed carrots. And we probably never expected, as adults, to be eating that same orange puree. But with the new trend of juicing and even an actual diet based on eating baby food, many people are doing just that. Although attempts to eat more vegetables, fruits, and whole grains are clearly based on good science, popular diets that encourage extreme behaviors—from raw foodism to colonics—are nothing more than pseudoscience.

The bottom line? Eating *more* raw vegetables is a lifestyle change; eating *only* raw vegetables is almost anorexia.

But I Don't Diet

These days, many of us carry a smartphone. Consider this: would you have purchased your current brand if it had a reputation for failing the vast majority of the time? Probably not.

But for years our society has kept dieting despite the well-documented failure rate.

Luckily for the weight-loss industry, dieters typically blame themselves when they gain the weight back, thus keeping their wallets open for the next miracle slimming plan. Some diets focus on a specific food—from grapefruit to cookies—while others, with the help of strategic exercise, promise to change a certain body part like your abs or backside. The tube-feeding diet, popularized in Europe, is so drastic that it requires a feeding tube that holds a minimal amount of liquid calories to be run through a person's nose right down into the stomach![1] Low-carbohydrate diets are popular worldwide from Atkins (in the United States) to Dukan (in France). Others encourage more obvious—though no more effective—approaches such as consuming very few calories per day or skipping meals. Some people jump on a certain diet bandwagon only to jump off and then start the same—or possibly different—one later. Unfortunately, as discussed in chapter 3, chronic or "yo-yo" dieting is typically associated with weight *gain*, rather than loss, over time.

You might be breathing a sigh of relief right now thinking, *But I don't diet.* Jenni used to believe the same thing even though she did restrict herself to small amounts of certain types of food due to concerns about her weight. That's clearly one form of dieting. She knows that now. As the public has become increasingly savvy to the mantra "Diets don't work," the diet industry has stayed in business by cleverly repackaging its wares as "lifestyle changes." Why else would they be promoting books with names like *The No Diet, Diet?*[2] Although some lifestyle changes are healthy, others can be dieting in disguise.

Here are just a few examples.

Food Allergies

Are you avoiding dairy or gluten because you think you might be allergic or intolerant? Food allergies involve a severe, possibly fatal, reaction to a limited number of foods—most commonly soy, wheat, eggs, milk, fish, shellfish, peanuts, or tree nuts. Studies suggest that approximately 6 percent of children and 1 to 2 percent of adults have *bona fide* food allergies[3] and must therefore abstain from at least one of these foods. Similarly, celiac disease, an autoimmune disorder that affects less than 1 percent of American adults, requires that sufferers follow a gluten-free diet and abstain from many types of foods and liquids, including wheat, French fries, soy sauce, and beer. Although food allergies are a very real phenomenon, in some cases they are just another smoke screen for dieting. A recent nationally representative study found that 96 percent of American adults who reported following a gluten-free diet tested negative for celiac disease via blood analysis.[4] Indeed, the National Institute of Allergy and Infectious Disease explicitly discourages food allergy self-diagnosis since people tend to be wrong in 50 to 90 percent of cases.[5] According to Klarman Eating Disorders Center dietitian Jaimie Winkler, "With a lot of food intolerances, people cite bloating and stomach discomfort as 'the symptom,' but truthfully, it's very human to sometimes bloat and have discomfort after meals. If it resolves within thirty minutes, chances are you aren't allergic, just human."[6] In light of these findings, we recommend asking your doctor for a skin test, blood test, or food challenge test before emptying your cupboards of bread, nuts, and pasta.

Sugar and Flour Addiction

A new generation of research on the possibility of food addiction has identified that anticipation of eating highly palatable food activates areas of the brain similar to those activated by drugs and alcohol.[7] Some—but not all—Twelve Step programs even ask their members to abstain from foods like sugar and white flour, which they believe are addictive.[8] But there is no evidence that eliminating specific foods (such as flour or sugar) from your diet is an effective way to prevent binge eating. On the contrary, there is much more evidence that trying to eliminate these foods from your diet will make you even *more* likely to binge. Here's why: we frequently crave what we won't let ourselves have. Have you ever turned down a dessert that you really wanted at a restaurant only to get home with an intense desire for something sweet? Dr. Thomas has worked with many patients who have exhausted their willpower trying to avoid eating a delicious homemade cookie at a party, only to feel deprived and binge on an entire box of stale store-bought cookies on the drive home.

Vegetarianism

There are all kinds of good reasons to become vegetarian (eating a plant-based diet without meat) or even vegan (abstaining from all animal products). Some are tied to long-standing cultural and religious beliefs; others stem from authentic concerns for animal rights. But some are just excuses for dieting. We have connected with many people who suffer from almost anorexia and other officially recognized eating disorders who say things like, "I can't eat that, because I'm a vegetarian," or "I would love to have a piece of your birthday cake; too bad

I'm vegan." If you are considering becoming vegetarian, it's important to be honest with yourself about your motivation for limiting your diet. In one study, 42 percent of vegetarian women who had previously been treated for an eating disorder identified weight management as their primary motivation for avoiding meat, compared to 0 percent of those with no eating disorder history.[9] So if you don't belong to any vegetarian organizations, have never read a book on factory farming, and wouldn't touch a vegan cupcake with a ten-foot pole, you may want to rethink your decision to go meat and/or dairy free.

Going "Raw"

For those who find that vegetarianism and veganism include far too many food choices, going "raw" takes restriction to the next level. Raw foodism is the practice of consuming only uncooked and unprocessed foods, such as fruits, vegetables, nuts, and seeds. Although it sounds healthy, research shows it may cause more harm than good. According to former raw foodist Frederic Patenaude, "Cravings for cooked food are the number one complaint raw foodists have."[10] He recalled in his book *Raw Food Controversies*, "One day, I was walking down the street, feeling this amazing craving for food. At that moment, I would have eaten anything: burgers, French fries, or even a steak. However, I didn't allow these thoughts into my consciousness. I was determined to keep eating 100% raw."[11] And in a large study of German adults who had consumed at least 70 percent of their diet as raw foods for at least two years, 38 percent were deficient in vitamin B12.[12] Given that B12 deficiency can cause a variety of physical and mental health problems—including fatigue, depression, and memory problems—you may want to think twice before opting to consume all of your foods at 118 degrees or lower.

Religious Restriction

Many people eat, or rather don't eat, in accordance with their religious views. Various forms of fasting are common practice in some religious traditions. For some, this is a way of life—tied to family roots and values—that truly works for them. But for others, spiritual beliefs become an excuse to restrict. We know many people with almost anorexia who have "given up" chocolate for Lent or who have fasted during Ramadan solely to lose weight. For example, as Cherry Boone O'Neill (daughter of American singer Pat Boone) recounted in her anorexia memoir *Starving for Attention*, "Fasting on Thanksgiving Day had really saved me. . . . When I was asked why I had not loaded up my plate like everyone else I just answered with spiritual overtones, 'I'm fasting today,' and that was that!"[13] But is it truly a sacrifice to give up chocolate or another food that you are already afraid to eat? When asked whether individuals with eating disorders should fast on Yom Kippur (the Jewish day of atonement), Orthodox rabbi Dovid Goldwasser responded, "I try to answer the spiritual conflict and say that no, God wants you to eat. Your eating on that day is considered as if you fasted."[14] Indeed, if you have almost anorexia, it makes more sense to challenge yourself by eating during these times of spiritual self-reflection.

Caloric Restriction for Longevity

Proponents of calorie restriction (CR) for longevity believe that consistently consuming 10 to 40 percent fewer calories per day than your body burns will make you live longer. Although early research on rats appeared to support this hypothesis, a 2012 study of rhesus monkeys (who are genetically more similar to humans) failed to find any difference in lifespan between those who were adequately fed versus those who were calorie-restricted.[15] Moreover, as clinical psychologist Kelly Vitousek has pointed out, rats and humans live very different lifestyles: "Laboratory animals are typically isolated in individual cages, protected or exempted from germs, temperature variation, work, fatigue, social interaction, parenting and competition. In effect, their only job is to cope with CR, so that all of the meager energy supplied by their otherwise optimal diets can be put straight to that purpose."[16] Think of it this way: if you are constantly hungry, irritable, and tired on a calorie-restricted diet, your life might just feel longer!

Jenni's Journey

I heard about caloric restriction for longevity in college when I was studying biochemistry. I remember a professor telling me about research on how semi-starved rats lived longer. And I distinctly remember thinking, *I guess I will live longer than others, because I semi-starve myself.* Ed loved this new information and repeatedly used it against me saying, "See, I told you. You *are* healthier than other people." In truth, I was very sick, and even if my diet was setting me up to live longer (it wasn't), I was miserable. Who wants to live longer in a state of misery? Not me. Not anymore.

Another Day, Another "–Rexia"

A disturbing new media trend is to use the tag "–rexia" to create popular labels, not official diagnoses. More times than not, cutesy terms like *brideorexia* are simply other words for almost anorexia and other officially recognized eating disorders. Unfortunately, fad –rexias give the false impression that eating disorders are not associated with real suffering. For example, Societal Ed might say, "Brideorexia isn't serious. It's just what every bride goes through before her big day." But if a bride really has anorexia, it is very serious, and it is definitely not cute. We describe just a handful of such terms next. By the time this book is in your hands, there will probably be even more.

Brideorexia

It's no secret that many brides feel pressure to look their best walking down the aisle. Pre-wedding weight loss is further normalized by popular television shows like *Bridal Bootcamp* and *Shedding for the Wedding*, which award dream nuptials to the contestant who loses the most. In one study of subscribers to a bridal expo mailing list, 70 percent of brides-to-be planned to lose weight for their wedding day—twenty-three pounds, on average. Some even reported using extreme behaviors such as skipping meals, fasting, and purging to achieve this goal.[17] But let's get real: crash dieting to fit into a wedding dress is a dangerous practice that could lead to a long-term marriage with Ed.

Orthorexia

In simplest terms, *orthorexia nervosa* is an unhealthy obsession with healthy eating. Rather than being preoccupied with food *quantity* (as in anorexia), individuals with orthorexia are preoccupied with food *quality* and may follow very restrictive eating plans in the misguided pursuit of a disease-free life. Individuals who become obsessed with so-called "clean eating" (such as avoiding white sugar, white flour, preservatives, and all other processed foods) might qualify as having orthorexia if their attempts seriously interfere with their quality of life. In addition to being vegan or eating a raw diet, some individuals try to prevent cancer by following a "macrobiotic" diet that avoids white carbohydrates and red meat, favoring brown rice, vegetables, fish, and sea vegetables. Alternative medicine physician Steven Bratman coined the term orthorexia nervosa (derived from the Greek terms *ortho* meaning "right" or "correct," and *rexia* meaning "hunger") in his seminal book *Health Food Junkies.* According to Bratman, there is a great deal of overlap between orthorexia and almost anorexia. An innocent desire to eat "healthier" can lead to a false sense of pride: *I am doing what others cannot. I am controlling my food.* Of course, the food is really controlling the eater when the undercover agenda is weight loss. By adopting a macrobiotic or raw diet, you can, according to Bratman, "'accidentally' live up to the Barbie image without admitting you believe in doing so."[18] But let's be clear: orthorexia can lead to nutritional deficiencies, social isolation, and, in some of Bratman's own patients, death.

Pregorexia

Women who feel uncomfortable with pregnancy-induced weight and body changes may strictly limit calorie intake, a phenomenon the media has termed "pregorexia."[19] Fueled in part by tabloid reports of super-svelte celebrities sporting the "perfect little baby bump" and famous "yummy mummies" who have "lost the baby weight!" at warp speed, new mothers have recently reported dangerous weight-loss behaviors as extreme as pumping and dumping breast milk to purge calo-ries.[20] We know that prenatal calorie restriction can lead to growth retardation and birth defects. The Dutch Famine Study showed that women who were pregnant between 1944 and 1946 in cities affected by famine had an increased risk of having a child with spina bifida, hydrocephalus, cerebral palsy, epilep-sy, or spastic diplegia at birth—and schizophrenia later in life— when compared to children born to mothers in cities not affected by the famine in those same years.[21] If you are an expecting mom, we strongly encourage you to follow the advice of your doctor—not the diet industry.

Drunkorexia

With binge drinking ubiquitous on today's college campuses, many young people worry about pouring on the pounds in the form of beer and cocktails. In a recent study, 39 percent of col-lege students reported restricting calories prior to consuming alcohol,[22] primarily to prevent weight gain and increase the speed of intoxication. Although it's true that alcohol is high in calories, drinking your dinner is not the solution to managing your weight. As with other fad "–rexias," don't let the cheeky term *drunkorexia* mislead you. The combination of disordered eating and alcohol abuse actually has more pernicious health consequences than either behavior in isolation. In this study, female students who restricted food, fat, or calorie intake on drinking days were more likely to report experiencing memory loss, being injured, being taken advantage of sexually, and having unprotected sex while drinking compared to those who did not restrict. Male students who restricted their diets on drinking days were more likely to get into physical fights.

• • •

What will be next? Pizzarexia? With all of the different labels and approaches to food, it is difficult to know what is real, what is good, and what is downright crazy. Whether you begin restricting your food as a lifestyle change or justify a radical regime by latching on to the next fad –rexia, dieting by any other name is still dieting. We were just kidding about pizzarexia, but if your next lifestyle change were gluten-free *and* vegan, you wouldn't be ordering delivery from Domino's anytime soon. And if you did break down and eat a forbidden slice, you might find yourself desperately trying to compensate for it, as we'll discuss next.

Almost Purging

In the 1988 dark comedy *Heathers*, which deals with high school popularity, one young woman says to the other as she emerges from the bathroom, "Grow up, Heather. Bulimia is so '87."[23] Just as *diet* is quickly becoming a four-letter word, public awareness campaigns are now successfully educating the public about the dangers of purging. Not only do vomiting, laxatives, and diuretics have harmful side effects; they are also an inefficient form of weight management. Laboratory studies of women with bulimia nervosa have found that the majority of binge calories are retained after either vomiting or taking laxatives.[24] Fortunately, longitudinal data suggest that the prevalence of bulimia nervosa has been steadily declining in the United States and the United Kingdom since the 1990s.[25]

Unfortunately, purging is still more common than you might think. While self-induced vomiting is probably the first example that comes to mind—followed by laxative and diuretic abuse—other more insidious practices currently recommended under the mantle of health are simply veiled attempts to compensate for calories. And they, too, can be dangerous. After all, juice fasting is still fasting, slimming teas are just herbal laxatives, and colonics are just fancy (not to mention pricey) enemas. And possibly the most deadly of all is medication misuse.

Juice Fasting

Some fasts are clearly marketed as diets. Take, for example, the fourteen-day lemonade fast that American singer Beyoncé Knowles purportedly followed to lose weight for her role in the movie *Dreamgirls*.[26] Others, however, claim that subsisting on liquefied fruit and vegetables (or nothing at all) for several days will cleanse and detoxify your body from past overindulgences (such as food, cigarettes, or alcohol). Here's the truth: fasting is a compensatory behavior recognized in the *DSM-5* as a symptom of bulimia nervosa. There are no proven detoxification benefits to fasting and no evidence that our bodies are even "toxic" to begin with. Not only do individuals report feeling hungry and fatigued while fasting, but only 18 percent of the ensuing weight loss is fat—the other 82 percent is water and muscle.[27] No wonder fasting doesn't help people lose weight in the long-term; even Beyoncé regained her famous curves when she ditched the lemonade.

Natural Herbs

When it comes to purging, herbs are the new craze. Although many of Dr. Thomas's patients still take laxatives and diuretics that are specifically marketed as such, others drink so-called slimming teas or take herbal weight-loss supplements. Dr.

Thomas's cross-cultural research with Dr. Anne Becker has demonstrated that, as far away as Fiji, adolescent girls are repurposing traditional herbs (that is, those typically used to promote health or fight against illness) to induce vomiting or diarrhea in the name of weight loss. Interestingly, Fijian girls who reported herbal purgative use exhibited levels of distress and impairment very similar to that of those who purged through vomiting and laxative use,[28] suggesting that herbs might not be as innocuous as people think. When Dr. Thomas gently points out to patients that such herbal products typically contain either laxative or diuretic ingredients (check the label), they usually defend the products as safe—after all, they are "natural." But let's face it: so is arsenic.

Colonics

Another purging trend recently popularized at spas across the United States and Europe is colonics. You may have heard it called colon cleansing, colon irrigation, or colon hydrotherapy. During a colonic, a colon hydrotherapist inserts a tube into the rectum, flushing the colon with water to expel the "sludge" caking the inside. Practitioners, who charge up to $100 for this service, claim that colonics promote detoxification and weight loss. What they might not tell you about is the possible side effects, which include cramping, bloating, nausea, dehydration, bowel perforation, and infection.[29] In reality, you don't need colonics to get rid of waste—your body already does this naturally. Plus, there is absolutely no "sludge" caking the lining of the colon, and there is zero evidence that colonics lead to long-term weight loss. By the time food material reaches your colon, most of the calories have already been absorbed.

Diabulimia

Individuals with type 1 diabetes sometimes purge by reducing or omitting insulin doses. Referred to as "eating disorder—diabetes mellitus type 1" by clinicians, you may have heard it called *diabulimia* in the popular press. When insulin doses are omitted, glucose accumulates in the blood and is excreted through urine, resulting in temporary weight loss. This dangerous behavior can result in devastating medical consequences, including loss of limbs, blindness, kidney damage, and even death. In one study, women with type 1 diabetes who reported insulin restriction had a three-fold increase in mortality risk over the eleven-year follow-up period. Among the deceased, insulin restrictors died an average of thirteen years earlier than non-insulin-restrictors.[30] If you have type 1 diabetes and are considering cutting back on your insulin to lose weight, please do not open this Pandora's box. If you are already doing this, contact your diabetes health care provider immediately. It could save your life.

• • •

The take-home message? Even if you aren't vomiting or taking laxatives, you are purging if you engage in any behavior designed to "make up for" food you've already eaten. At best, you are wasting time and money on an ineffective and potentially harmful weight-loss strategy. At worst, you may have almost anorexia or an officially recognized eating disorder.

Jenni's Journey

I don't make myself throw up, I thought, while reading an information pamphlet about bulimia, *so I must not have an eating disorder.* This particular piece of paper included numerous facts about the dangers of throwing up, but I didn't see anything about what I was doing. At that point, I was bingeing a lot but not throwing up at all. In response to a binge, Ed would say, "Since you can't seem to handle food, Jenni, just don't eat."

So, I would fast, and in our society, that is something that can bring you accolades. I still can't believe how many compliments I received for having an eating disorder: *You have such control. I wish I could eat like you.* Now I know that fasting can be very destructive. In fact, fasting and excessive exercise (both of which are nonpurging compensatory behaviors) are in the same category of danger as more well-known purging behaviors.

With support and time, I was finally able to stop fasting altogether; looking back, I can't imagine how I was once able to deprive myself of food for such long periods of time. I don't miss having that ability, but instead, I look back with sadness. I missed out on a lot of life because I was starving. My family sometimes talks about fun memories that I simply don't recall, not because they didn't happen, but because my malnourished brain had trouble remembering things long-term.

If you battle excessive restricting, try not to believe the compliments that you might be receiving. What's really happening is that, with each calorie not eaten, you are damaging your body and missing out on life. Make a decision to work toward getting on track with food, and get your life back in the process.

Camille

Camille was forty-two years old when her father died of pancreatic cancer. Feeling lost and bereaved, she became increasingly aware of her own mortality. If Camille were to pass away, who would take care of her ten-year-old son, Mason? *Certainly not my deadbeat ex-husband,* she thought. *He's been behind on his child support payments since the divorce, and he hasn't attended a single one of Mason's soccer games this year.*

In an attempt to channel her anxiety into action, Camille began taking steps to improve her family's health. Her first dietary changes were sensible. She cut back on processed foods and started eating a more colorful diet rich in fruits and vegetables. She even got Mason to try new whole grains like millet, amaranth, and quinoa. One night while perusing cancer prevention information online, she stumbled upon a blog about macrobiotics. Fascinated by the potential power of food to heal her body and prevent disease, she began visiting the site every day. Was she ready to sign up for the disease-free life promised by this ancient Japanese dietary practice? Yes, please! With enthusiasm, she emptied her refrigerator of eggplant, potatoes, and peppers (too "yin," according to the blog) and stopped buying chicken and eggs (apparently too "yang"). Increasingly hypervigilant for possible signs of disease, Camille noticed that her stomach felt upset after eating cheese or yogurt. Since macrobiotics discouraged dairy consumption anyway, she decided to cut these out. Besides, she'd always suspected that she might be lactose intolerant.

Strangely, the more foods she cut out of her diet, the better she felt about herself. As her newfound macrobiotic lifestyle became increasingly important to her identity, Camille's healthy eating guidelines crystallized into rigid rules. At Mason's birthday party, she felt incredibly guilty for indulging in a small slice of cake. In penance for going off-plan, she drank two cups of herbal slimming tea that night—to help the toxins pass through her system more quickly. She didn't want those carcinogenic substances inside of her for long—she might develop pancreatic cancer, like her dad did.

She was faced with temptation once again at Mason's year-end soccer banquet, which was catered by a local pizza parlor. At Mason's urging, she took a few bites of a BBQ chicken pie. She immediately wished she hadn't. Overcome with panic, she could almost feel the tumors metastasizing inside her body. She barely made it to the women's room before throwing up. Although she hadn't meant to vomit, she was surprised when a sense of calm washed over her. The pizza was out of her system. Her body had ejected the impurity. It somehow seemed totally reasonable, like the time she gave Mason an emergency emetic after he accidentally ingested cleaning fluid as a toddler.

Soon, Camille was vomiting after eating normal amounts of food about once or twice per week. It was a handy way to compensate for going off plan, and it certainly helped her follow her macrobiotic practice despite constant encouragement to cheat by eating turkey (on Thanksgiving), French fries (when she took Mason for fast food), or white pasta (on a date at an Italian restaurant). And she considered her slight weight loss, which she did not realize was simply due to dehydration, a nice side effect. *Not only will being thin reduce cancer risk*, she thought, *but with all of this extra male attention I'm getting, maybe I'll find Mason a dad after all.*

Camille started worrying about her eating behavior, however, when she noticed her post-meal stomach pain intensifying. Concerned that she might have a medical problem, she visited a gastrointestinal specialist to investigate. She tried to calm herself by reading a macrobiotic magazine in the waiting room and couldn't help but think how unfair it would be if she got cancer despite her valiant dietary efforts. Fortunately, after visiting four different physicians and undergoing several invasive tests, she received a clean bill of health. In fact, she was still at a normal—although low—weight, and she wasn't lactose intolerant after all.

Without a physical cause for her pain, Camille wondered if it might be psychological. *No, it just can't be,* she thought. *I would never have the time to deal with something like that.* As a single working mom with an already too-busy schedule, she did her best to dismiss the idea. Ironically, Camille had been quite willing to devote a significant number of hours to getting all of those physical tests. Needing psychological help was just unfamiliar to her—and thus very scary. But, as more time passed, Camille had to admit that she had long since started to feel confused about whether her vomiting episodes continued to be involuntary. For example, she had noticed that the high likelihood that she would vomit in the evenings gave her "permission" to eat non-macrobiotic foods that she wouldn't normally allow herself to have. Now that she'd purchased new clothes in her new, smaller size, she worried that if she stopped vomiting they would no longer fit. But she was more concerned—yet again—about what would happen to Mason if she weren't around. Despite the positive medical report, she couldn't shake this strange feeling that all of her throwing up might physically hurt her. Hands shaking, she clicked away from the macrobiotic website and typed something new into her search engine: "Is making yourself throw up an eating disorder?"

Your Own Relationship with Food

DSM-5 might classify Camille's eating behavior as purging disorder (since she purges but does not binge eat), whereas Steven Bratman might call it orthorexia. In either case, her behaviors are certainly almost anorexic. Are yours? You might be doing something with food that you have never seen described in a book (even this one). You might think that you are the only person in the world doing what you are doing. Ed will proclaim that you are extremely special in your eating-disordered behaviors. (You are certainly unique as a person but not for your eating disorder.)

If Ed can convince you that no one else is doing what you do with food, then he can hold you hostage saying, "No one will understand you. I am the only one who 'gets' you, so stick with me." But Ed is lying. How can you tell? He opened his mouth! Other people, possibly ones reading this very book right now, are doing the same thing with food as you. Some people, like Emma, whom you met in chapter 2, even have seemingly random rules like always eating even numbers of foods (for example, eight raisins rather than seven) and eating clockwise around each plate. To mask feelings of hunger, others abuse substances, such as cigarettes, sugar-free gum, coffee, or diet soda. (Diet Dr. Pepper sales probably took a hit when Jenni recovered.) Although cigarettes are certainly harmful, we do not believe that there is anything inherently wrong with a stick of gum, your favorite latte, or Diet Coke. But we'd like you to be really honest with yourself about your motives.

At first it was difficult for Camille to acknowledge that shape and weight played a role in her dietary rules and purging behaviors. But writing them out on paper helped her identify multiple motives (table 4). Using table 5 or in a notebook, describe any dietary rules that you are attempting to follow and any methods you are currently using to try to compensate for food you have already eaten. If you don't think you are trying to follow any rules, ask yourself whether you would feel guilty for eating differently than you currently do. For example, if eating an evening snack would send you into a tailspin of self-recrimination, you might have an implicit rule about eating only three meals per day. Then comes the hard part—examining your rationale for each behavior. First write down what you tell yourself (or others). Next, write down any possible, more eating-disordered, alternatives. Of course, there can be many reasons behind a single eating behavior, and they each differ from person to person. But chances are good that if you are reading this book, you realize that you have (or that a loved one has) a problem with food. That realization is a huge milestone. If you have already taken that important step, we encourage you to get the most out of this book: be as honest as you can with the exercise that follows. Jenni ultimately found that the secrets she kept, especially from herself, kept her sick.

Table 4.

Camille's Dietary Rules and Purging Behaviors

This table shows Camille's answers to these questions.

DIETING		
What dietary rules do I try to follow that require me to actively restrict my caloric intake, fast all day, or avoid specific foods (suspected allergens, sugar, flour, meat, dairy, or cooked foods)?		
Describe each dietary rule:	**Why do I say I do this?**	**Why might I *really* be doing this?**
1. I must eat a macrobiotic diet.	1. I don't want to get cancer like my dad.	1. I want to lose weight.
2. I can't eat any dairy.	2. I think I might be lactose intolerant.	2. Cheese on the lips, cheese on the hips.
3. Potatoes are off limits.	3. Macrobiotics says they are unhealthy.	3. Carbohydrates will make me fat.
PURGING		
How do I compensate for past dietary "indulgences"? (Include vomiting, laxatives, diuretics, fasting—including juice fasting—detoxification, herbs, slimming teas, enemas, colon cleansing, and anything else.)		
Describe each purging behavior:	**Why do I say I do this?**	**Why might I *really* be doing this?**
1. Drink slimming tea	1. I want the toxins to pass through my body more quickly.	1. Birthday cake will undo all of my hard work trying to lose weight.
2. Throw up my food	2. Non-macro foods upset my stomach.	2. I feel really guilty for eating pizza.

Table 5.
Your Dietary Rules and Purging Behaviors

Now answer these questions for yourself.

DIETING		
What dietary rules do I try to follow that require me to actively restrict my caloric intake, fast all day, or avoid specific foods (suspected allergens, sugar, flour, meat, dairy, or cooked foods)?		
Describe each dietary rule:	**Why do I say I do this?**	**Why might I really be doing this?**
1.	1.	1.
2.	2.	2.
3.	3.	3.

PURGING		
How do I compensate for past dietary "indulgences"? (Include vomiting, laxatives, diuretics, fasting—including juice fasting—detoxification, herbs, slimming teas, enemas, colon cleansing, and anything else.)		
Describe each purging behavior:	**Why do I say I do this?**	**Why might I really be doing this?**
1.	1.	1.
2.	2.	2.
3.	3.	3.

This table can be downloaded at www.almostanorexic.com.

Almost Anorexia in Sheep's Clothing

The list of ways that people approach food is endless. Conveniently for Ed, many contemporary trends allow individuals to diet and purge without acknowledging it. This can make almost anorexia and other officially recognized eating disorders increasingly difficult to detect—in a loved one, and even in yourself. Stay tuned for chapter 7, where we'll provide strategies for normalizing your eating and systematically addressing the dietary rules and purging behaviors that may keep you imprisoned. But first, let's turn to the issue that might underlie your desire to go gluten-free or detoxify with a juice fast: your relationship with your body.

| 5 |

Optical Illusions
Your Relationship with Your Body

Most of us feel dissatisfied with our appearance at one time or another. But individuals with almost anorexia and other officially recognized eating disorders often feel so unhappy with their shape or weight that it distorts not only the way they see their body but their entire life as well. Today, when Jenni looks back at photographs of herself when she was underweight, she can see that she was entirely too thin, her hair was dull, and her eyes looked tired and sad. But back then, she perceived a different image altogether. Wearing "Ed glasses," as she sometimes says, Jenni noticed just the "fat" body parts that Ed wanted her to see. Only when she finally took off these eating-disordered glasses could she see the truth. Like the ones your doctor might prescribe, Ed glasses come in all strengths and styles. Are you wearing a pair? Is your loved one?

The Unattainable Ideal

Tell me the truth—do I look fat in this? . . . I should really work out more. . . . Ugh—she really shouldn't be wearing that. This is fat talk. We've all heard it, and most of us have engaged in it at one time or another. Anthropologist Mimi Nichter coined the term "fat talk" in her 2001 book of the same name.[1] Sadly, people often connect around the language of fat. A memorable scene from the teen comedy *Mean Girls*[2] involves three girls standing in front of a mirror critiquing themselves: the first pokes at her "huge" hips, the second "hates" her calves, and the third laments her "man shoulders." When they finally turn to the fourth girl, who is at a loss for body criticism, the original three roll their eyes in disbelief. Contemporary body image ideals are so unattainable—for women and men alike—that those who *don't* take part in social self-deprecation are often considered abnormal.

Supermodel: The Feminine Ideal

We all know that society's ideal woman—from Barbie dolls to supermodels—is typically represented as tall, thin, toned, tan, young, and blond. And with such a dizzying array of methods to enhance female appearance—plastic surgery, Botox, anti-aging products, and makeup—there's always an opportunity for something to look wrong. It's no wonder, then, that in one study, 50 percent of girls ages three to six said that they "sometimes" or "almost always" worried about being fat.[3] And although there is less pressure on ethnic minority women, such as African Americans and Latinas, to be extremely thin,[4] societal expectations for them to have an hourglass figure with round breasts and buttocks—à la singer Jennifer Lopez—can be just as oppressive.

Superman: The Masculine Ideal

Men, too, are under increasing pressure to go from Clark Kent to Superman, ditching "scrawny arms," "pot bellies," or "man boobs" for six-pack abs and chiseled biceps. Even young boys' action figures sport supersized bodies—with waists and biceps of the same size—that could not be obtained in real life without steroids. Distinctive body ideals for males may help explain why some men with almost anorexia are terrified of being too big, while others are terrified of being too small.[5] Some even struggle with muscle dysmorphia—a preoccupation with being insufficiently lean and muscular, leading to a diet or workout schedule that interferes with psychosocial functioning.[6] Though not technically an eating disorder, muscle dysmorphia is a sub-type of body dysmorphic disorder that affects both males and females and often co-occurs with eating disorders. Individuals with body dysmorphic disorder worry excessively about aspects of their appearance broader than just shape or weight (from receding hairlines to crooked noses) but share the crippling self-perception of imagined ugliness that plagues those with almost anorexia.[7]

In *The Adonis Complex*, psychiatrist Harrison Pope and colleagues have discussed how body image problems can be even more insidious in males because worrying about appearance and discussing feelings have historically been considered female concerns. This leaves men "trapped between impossible ideals on the one side and taboos against feeling and talking on the other."[8] And it might be even worse for some subgroups. Research suggests that gay men are even more likely to be dissatisfied with their bodies than their heterosexual counterparts.[9] Licensed marriage and family therapist Brad Kennington, who specializes in treating males with eating disorders, told us, "Gay men are under the same pressures that straight women are to achieve the so-called perfect body. After all, they are both trying to attract men as potential mates. Having the ideal body (toned, fit, youthful looking) in the gay community provides gay men with power, status, and prestige."[10]

Not Even Models Look Like Models

Supermodel Cindy Crawford famously told *Redbook*, "Even I don't wake up looking like Cindy Crawford! What people see on magazine covers is one moment that was perfect—the wind, the light, the hair, the makeup. That's a two-hour process."[11] We don't know about you, but we certainly don't wake up with a team of professionals around us. Increasingly, however, not even the wind, light, hair, and makeup that Crawford describes is sufficient to make models look like models. Today, society's perfect 10 is simply not attainable without photo manipulation software like Photoshop.

Digital artist Roy A. Cui has retouched covers for fashion, entertainment, and lifestyle magazines. Cui told us that, when a retoucher receives an image from a photographer, there is an "unspoken" preliminary list of perceived flaws to correct. This list includes

- eliminating flyaway hairs
- fixing skin (blemishes, bags and/or dark rings under the eyes, freckles, creases in neck and armpits, *any* sign of cellulite)
- minimizing signs of aging (age spots, wrinkles by the eyes and mouth, veins in hands and feet)
- whitening eyes and teeth

- smoothing wrinkles in clothing
- using the Photoshop "liquefy" filter to shape the waist, bust, arms, hips, and thighs to smooth bulges and shape the subject's silhouette

But it's still not over. Cui continued, "Then the photographer will usually request additional changes and forward the files to their client (magazine editor, art director) for final approval. There might even be more changes from their client after that."[12]

To see an example of how retouching, makeup, hair, and wind are used together to transform someone into a glamorous billboard model, check out the seventy-five-second "Dove Evolution" video, which went viral on YouTube in 2006. And for a real-life story: New York model Sara Ziff, who has been the face of advertising campaigns for Tommy Hilfiger and Kenneth Cole, told us that once her own mother did not recognize her on the face of a billboard just blocks away from her childhood home.[13]

Furthermore, some magazine editors have recently admitted to engaging in "reverse retouching"—reshaping certain painfully thin models to look healthier by filling in gaunt cheeks and erasing jutting collar bones, while still preserving their slender silhouettes. According to former British *Cosmopolitan* editor Leah Hardy, "Thanks to retouching, our readers—and those of *Vogue*, *Self*, and *Healthy* magazine— never saw the horrible, hungry downside of skinny. That these underweight girls don't look glamorous in the flesh. Their skeletal bodies, dull, thinning hair, spots and dark circles under their eyes were magicked away by technology, leaving only the allure of coltish limbs and Bambi eyes. A vision of perfection that simply didn't exist."[14] Tragically, this unreal image can kill. Both Brazilian model Ana Carolina Reston and French model Isabelle Caro died of complications related to anorexia nervosa in 2006 and 2010, respectively. More recently, in 2012, British model Bethaney Wallace died of anorexia.[15]

And the potentially negative impact of reverse retouching on readers' own body images isn't lost on Hardy, who has since admitted to feeling guilty about the practice: "No wonder women yearn to be super-thin when they never see how ugly thin can be," she said.[16] Of course, we are not implying that all thin people look bad. What we are saying is that forcing your body to be unnaturally thin for your size is obviously not going to be your best look. We truly look best when we are healthy and happy. If a voice in your head is disagreeing with that last sentence, consider that it just might be Societal Ed talking. (Too bad we can't just ask Roy Cui to Photoshop Ed's mouth shut.)

The ability to analyze and evaluate the media messages that we receive is crucial to developing a positive body image. Even if you know that images have been altered, it's helpful to remind yourself of this fact—and frequently. The human condition is one of forgetfulness. In one study, adding a label that said "Warning: These images have been digitally altered" prevented women from becoming dissatisfied with their own bodies after viewing a twelve-page fashion spread, compared to a no-label control condition which produced the predictable bump in body dissatisfaction.[17] Dr. Thomas tries to give patients a visual reminder of such altering in her body image group. She invites them to flick through fashion magazines, ripping out and crumpling up any pages featuring extremely underweight or drastically retouched models. They are inevitably surprised to see the heaping pile of crinkled images in the middle of the room at the end of the task. The magazines themselves have almost nothing left inside. Try it yourself.

Everyone Is Watching

Unfortunately, we are not the only ones who criticize our bodies. Increasingly, we live in a world that watches our weight. Melbourne's *Herald Sun* dubbed Australian swimmer Leisel Jones too fat to compete just days before she earned a silver medal for her country at the 2012 Olympic games.[18] New York City ballerina Jenifer Ringer, who has been open about her history of anorexia, appeared on the *Today* show to respond to a dance critic who accused her of having eaten "one sugarplum too many" before performing in *The Nutcracker*.[19] And British singer Adele didn't sit idly by when designer Karl Lagerfeld called her fat: "I've never wanted to look like models on the cover of magazines," she told *People*. "I represent the majority of women and I'm very proud of that."[20]

Today's world continuously looks at our bodies and judges. Most of us don't get to fire back in *People* after receiving a bad body review. This is especially true for children. Throughout their school years, kids who are larger are sometimes bullied, and children who are naturally skinny get teased too. Anyone who doesn't fit neatly into the middle—or closer to the thin side—can easily be on the receiving end of a negative comment. Indeed, regardless of BMI, weight-related teasing in childhood predicts the onset of disordered-eating behaviors in adolescence.[21] Unfortunately, this mentality stays the same as we grow older. Both teenagers and adults, for instance, can feel pressured to look "just right" to get a date or attract a mate. When Jenni signed up for an online dating site, she was surprised when it encouraged her to include at least one full-body photograph in her profile and required her to check a single box describing her body type as "athletic and toned," "about average," "curvy," or "heavyset." We are waiting for the media to coin the term *Matchorexia* for people who go on rigid weight-loss programs in the aftermath of creating an online dating profile. As an eating disorder therapist, Dr. Thomas also receives unsolicited feedback about her average-size body. A patient recently told her, "I feel like I can accept body image advice from you, because you are obviously comfortable carrying a few extra pounds." Another said, "You'll never understand what it's like to be me, because you are so thin." As a young clinician, Dr. Thomas once believed that her BMI needed to land exactly in the middle of the normal range to work with patients who have eating disorders (who tend to take particular note of their treatment provider's shape, as indicated). But Dr. Thomas soon realized that she would be most effective as a therapist not at a particular weight, but instead when she was taking best care of herself.

With the Internet constantly at our fingertips on smart-phones, laptops, and tablets, body bashing has grown to a whole new level. Making snide, witty comments about another person's body—known as bodysnarking—is commonplace and seemingly accepted. Blogs, Facebook, and other social media sites give all of us an avenue to comment publicly about not only celebrities but also the person we ran into at last night's party. Digital cameras on mobile phones turn most of us into potential paparazzi. With one click, a picture can be uploaded to Facebook for all to see. And this, in fact, seems to be fueling a "camera ready" mentality among ordinary people. In one study, 44 percent of Facebook users ages sixteen to forty said that when attending social events, they are always conscious that photos of them might get posted.[22] But while most of us are able to bounce back from *bodysnarking* or surreptitiously "de-tag" ourselves from unflattering photos (that is, remove the picture from our online profile), those with almost anorexia and other officially recognized eating disorders may perceive almost any comment about their bodies as utterly crushing to their overall self-esteem. Unfortunately, that was true for Dante.

Dante

A bead of sweat dripped onto Dante's copy of *Men's Health* magazine. He looked at his watch. *Just twenty more seconds before my next bench press set.* He shook the damp arm of his sweatshirt. Though he felt overheated in his baggy tracksuit, he was too embarrassed to wear a sleeveless shirt in front of the more muscular lifters. *When I lose enough body fat*, he promised himself.

On the walk to the locker room after his punishing two-hour workout, Dante gazed intently at his shape in the floor-to-ceiling gym mirror. *Am I getting bigger?* he wondered. The mental measurements he took every morning suggested that he was indeed adding inches, but Dante often worried that he was gaining fat, not muscle. No matter how carefully he watched his diet—which now consisted mainly of shakes, gels, and powders—he was never sure he'd perfected his carb-to-protein ratio. He made a mental note to pick up more creatine and fat-burning pills at the health food store later.

Spending less than a minute in the locker room, Dante grabbed his gym bag and avoided making eye contact with anyone before quietly slipping out. His wife, Joanna, wrinkled her nose when Dante hopped into the car. "You smell like a dirty sock," she teased. "Why don't you ever shower after working out those big muscles of yours?" Dante laughed, relieved that she was in a good mood after he had chosen to lift weights rather than accompanying her to a friend's party—yet again. He never showered or changed at the gym, for fear the other men would judge him as too flabby. And although Joanna was always complimenting his cut and toned body, Dante knew she was just being nice. *She has to say that*, he thought. *She's my wife.*

That evening, Dante and Joanna shared a relaxing dinner. Well, Joanna did at least. Dante didn't find meals particularly enjoyable; he much preferred just sticking to his shakes and supplements. In fact, Dante rarely ate actual meals except with Joanna, who always begged him to sit down at the table with her, especially on the nights before he went out of town for sales meetings.

"Water, no ice," he said to the flight attendant on the early morning flight. He needed some more water to mix with his breakfast shake to make it just right. The man sitting next to him, who was in his early thirties—around Dante's age— noticed and said, "Is that how you stay in such good shape?" Dante smiled, thinking, *Maybe my hard work is paying off.* "Nutrition and working out," Dante said. The man continued, "Would you mind sharing your workout routine with me? My girlfriend has been begging me to get fit—but not too buff— like you. She doesn't like really big muscles."

Dante felt like he'd been kicked in the stomach. *I knew it. Joanna has been lying.* He mumbled a response, then immediately put on his headphones, opened his laptop, and didn't talk for the rest of the flight. Although Dante usually prepared for sales presentations during flights, this time he decided to connect to the onboard Wi-Fi to try to figure out what he might be doing wrong at the gym. With just a few clicks on the Internet, he got his answer: steroids. *Why hadn't I thought of that before?* Dante believed that if he could just get bigger, everything would be okay. His newfound obsession with studying up on steroids and trying to figure out where to buy them interfered with his presentation that afternoon. Dante was originally hired for his energetic speaking style, but now his boss, Robert, couldn't help but notice his change in demeanor. This particular sales pitch was so bad that Robert planned to discuss it after all of their clients had cleared the room.

"Are things all right?" Robert asked. "Is everything okay with you and Joanna?" Dante responded, "Sure. I just don't see her that much. I'm so busy with work." *And working out,* Dante thought. Noticing Dante's blank stare, Robert could see that he wasn't going to get anywhere with this conversation and made a mental note to speak with the human resources department when they returned to the office. He knew that something wasn't right.

Walking back to his hotel room, Dante stewed over Robert's questioning. He had always prided himself on being a stellar employee. But recognizing that his presentation hadn't gone over well and that his last few talks hadn't been up to par, Dante wondered why he might be losing his edge. He thought about it all the way up the ten flights of stairs he ran to reach his top-floor suite. His in-flight magazine had indicated that stair stepping is helpful for building up calf muscles. Upon entering his room, he mindlessly flipped on the television just as an entertainment news show was mentioning a young female celebrity's suspected battle with anorexia. *I just don't understand. How can girls do that to themselves?* he wondered. *I take such great care of my body.*

How Do You Evaluate Yourself?

Dante did not have anorexia, but he did have an unspecified feeding and eating disorder that was interfering with both work and relationships. If almost all of us are exposed to an unattainable body image ideal, then why do only some, like Dante, develop almost anorexia? The answer lies, in part, in the relative importance of shape and weight to our self-esteem.

All of us have a system for judging ourselves. If we meet the standards we set in important life domains—from relationships to school—we feel successful. If not, we feel like we've failed. For example, Dr. Thomas's work is very important to her sense of self, so she is delighted when one of her scientific papers gets accepted for publication but frustrated when a research grant does not get funded. Clinical psychologist Josie Geller developed the pie chart tool that follows to help people work out which arenas of life are most important to them.[23]

Take a look at Dante's example in figure 6, and then try the exercise for yourself. We have listed common domains (such as relationships, work, and hobbies), but you should select only those that feel important to you, and feel free to add any additional ones. After you decide which areas are most important for you, assign them each a piece of the pie. (You can do this by writing in figure 7 or in a notebook, or by downloading the exercise at www.almostanorexic.com). The size of each slice should be determined by its relative significance to your self-esteem. Basing your self-esteem mainly (or even exclusively) on shape and weight is often referred to as the "core psychopathology" of eating disorders.[24] Indeed, research suggests that allocating a larger slice of the pie to shape and weight goes hand in hand with more severe disordered-eating behaviors and even predicts the onset of new such behaviors.[25] People with a healthy body image might not always like what they see in the mirror, but they do not base their entire self-worth on this. Both in our thirties, we don't particularly like that we still sometimes get pimples, but we don't base our self-worth on a blemish or two—or three. As you can see, for Dante, the domain most important to his self-esteem is muscularity (that is, a specific aspect of shape and weight). As psychiatrist Christopher Fairburn has pointed out, having a single slice dominate your pie chart is "risky" because "it is like having all your eggs in one basket."[26] In other words, it is great if you feel you are succeeding in that arena, but devastating if you feel you are not. When Dante believes that he is muscular enough, for example, he feels extremely confident, but when he feels flabby or scrawny, he is crushed. Another problem with allocating most of your self-esteem to weight and shape is that it makes other previously valued domains (like relationships or other talents) start to feel less important. This was certainly true for Dante, who rarely dined with his wife and started having difficulties at work.

Figure 6.

Dante's Self-Evaluation Pie Chart

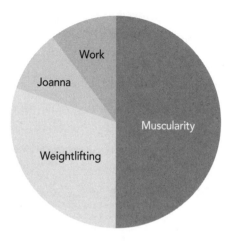

Now think about your own life. Which domains of your life have to be going well for you to feel good about yourself? Consider these:

- friends
- family
- work/school
- hobbies/talents
- romantic relationship
- shape/weight
- eating
- other(s)?

Using these domains, draw a pie chart so that the size of each slice is proportional to its importance to your self-esteem. Domains with larger slices are more important; those with smaller slices are less so.

Figure 7.
Your Self-Evaluation Pie Chart

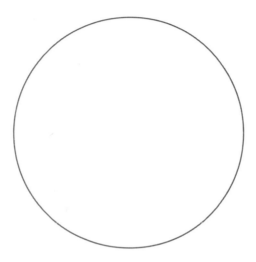

Wearing Ed Glasses

Basing much of your self-esteem on shape and weight causes you to view the world through Ed glasses. Eye-tracking research suggests that when individuals with almost anorexia and other officially recognized eating disorders look at photos of themselves, they tend to spend more time looking at body parts that they think are "ugly" than parts they think are "beautiful."[27] Hyperfocusing on perceived flaws, they tend to formulate an overall judgment of themselves that is both harsh and critical, and they later recall and ruminate about these imperfections. Once they have developed this critical view of their bodies, it can be difficult to change.

To illustrate this concept, take a look at the ambiguous picture created for this book by artist Emily Wierenga in figure 8. (You can also download this figure at www.almostanorexic.com.) Do you see a thin or a large woman? The figure is designed to be either one. If at first you see the larger woman whose body is positioned sideways facing to the right, it may be difficult for you to change your perspective and to see the thin woman whose body is facing forward with her head tilted up toward the left. To help you distinguish between the two, note that the thin woman's nose is raised higher, more smugly, and is actually the ear of the larger woman, who appears melancholy with her arms folded across her chest. The feather hat on the upper left belongs to the thin woman and also serves as a ponytail for the large woman. Wierenga, who herself recovered from anorexia nervosa and coauthored the body image book *Mom in the Mirror*,[28] designed the thin woman's regal robe to represent the large woman's layers of flesh. She told us, "In a society that equates thin with beauty and beauty with love, we long to be thin, and so we hide. Beneath layers of guilt and shame, not seeing ourselves for the royalty that we are."[29]

Just like the thin/large woman, our own bodies can be ambiguous figures—one day looking slim and svelte, the next day covered in rolls of fat. Unfortunately, it is all too easy to let this image dictate whether we should feel pride (like the thin woman) or shame (like the large woman). You may have found that, once you started seeing the ambiguous picture one way (that is, as either thin or fat), it was difficult for you to change perspectives. Just as you can get locked in to viewing the ambiguous figure one way, individuals with almost anorexia get locked in to viewing themselves as "fat." Their perception can be difficult to change, mainly because they begin to engage in behaviors that serve to maintain their negative self-view. As in a game of hide-and-seek, those with almost anorexia often alternate between avoidance, which is a desperate attempt to hide perceived flaws, and body checking, which is near-constant vigilance for any weight and shape changes.

Figure 8.

Thin or Large Woman?

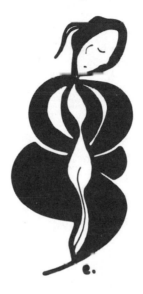

Created by Emily Wierenga
Available at www.almostanorexic.com

Are You Hiding Your Body?

A negative relationship with your body can be like living in a prison whose rules dictate what you can and cannot do. *Don't let anyone take your photo until you lose weight. Don't go to that party, because you look horrible in dress clothes.* Those with almost anorexia and other officially recognized eating disorders are significantly more likely than healthy individuals to engage in avoidance behaviors, such as refusing to be weighed, averting their eyes as they walk past reflective surfaces, and wearing baggy clothes to disguise their shape.[30] Avoidance behaviors can be subtle, such as making yourself sit or stand in a certain way that you think will make you appear thinner—whether in photos or in real life. These behaviors can be incredibly impairing too. Dr. Thomas has worked with patients who dress in the dark, rarely shower, or won't even get out of bed on "fat" days.

For example, Dante wore oversized sweatshirts at the gym and wouldn't shower or undress in the locker room, because he was worried that others would judge him negatively. Similarly, when Jenni first gained weight in recovery, she only wore—or hid out in—big, baggy clothes. A waistband pressing against her stomach seemed to scream out, *You need to lose some weight*, and pants that fit snugly against her hips said, *You're nothing special*. A friend once asked, "Are you ever going to wear jeans again?" Jenni responded that she could live her entire life without jeans. And she could have. But when we are slaves to our closets, we are not living a fulfilled life. Gratefully, Jenni kept learning and growing. Today, if you see her give a talk at your local university, you will most likely see her wearing a comfy pair of jeans.

Are You Checking Your Body?

Although seemingly different from body hiding, body checking is actually the opposite side of the same coin—the coin of basing your self-esteem primarily on shape and weight. When Jenni was struggling, she knew exactly how her clothes were "supposed" to fit. She pinched rolls of perceived fat—it was skin—on her stomach. She checked (and double-checked) to make sure that her thighs didn't touch at the top. During early recovery, she thought that getting rid of her scale might end the obsession with needing to know her exact weight. And it did.

Yet her struggle with body checking was nowhere near from over. No longer able to hop on the scale every morning, she began trying on a special pair of jeans, her new metric of thin and fat. The number on the size tag became her new obsession. Body checking behaviors like pinching your upper arms to measure fatness, seeing if your thighs spread when you sit down, and scrutinizing yourself in mirrors (or shop windows, or other people's sunglasses!) are common among women who struggle with disordered eating.[31] Men's checking behaviors more often revolve around muscularity, such as checking muscle definition in their abs, comparing the size of their chest and shoulders with others', or flexing their biceps in the mirror.[32] Like Dante, some measure their muscles to see how many inches they've gained or lost. Both males and females might compare their size and shape to that of other people.

Body checking can even occur outside of conscious awareness. Dr. Thomas once interviewed a patient who adamantly denied body checking, while simultaneously running her fingers along her clavicle, feeling for bone. Indeed, checking is so pervasive among individuals with almost anorexia that Dr. Thomas has even observed it in a blind patient whom she was treating. The patient shared that, "I do all of the checking, but without the eyes."[33] Undeterred by her lack of sight, this young woman repeatedly felt for bony protrusions in her face, ribcage, spine, and hips. During conversations with others, she attempted to estimate their height through voice location and weight through voice pitch, with higher locations indicating taller height and lower pitch indicating greater abdominal girth. Her need to engage in body comparisons—even approximate ones—was that strong! Ultimately, she learned to apply her ingenuity and imagination to a more worthy goal: applying to graduate school.

But I Don't Care about Shape or Weight

Although body image disturbance is an extremely common feature of almost anorexia and other officially recognized eating disorders, it is by no means universal. There are some individuals who, despite low body weight, do not endorse a fear of fatness.[34] As we mentioned previously, anorexia without fear

Jenni's Journey

The mirror told me all kinds of things. It sometimes said that I was thin. Other times, when I was scrutinizing my body, it made clear that I was thin with the exception of _____. (Fill in the blank with a body part of choice.) Even when the mirror said that I was skinny, I still wasn't happy because I was too busy worrying about what *might* happen. *What if I put on pounds?* And I did, in fact, gain some weight in the healing process. At that point, every time I looked in the mirror, I saw a fat person staring back at me, so I tried to avoid my reflection as much as possible. Mostly, I just closed my eyes around any and all mirrors. I became an expert at getting around in public restrooms with my eyes closed. That was how much I hated my body. Although challenging, my relationship with my body eventually changed. I learned to pay attention to my whole self when I looked in the mirror—I was no longer just a collection of body parts. I can finally say that I love my body! When I look in the mirror today, I like what I see. If I am tired or stressed out, I might not like what I see as well as on other days. Or if someone has recently made a comment to me about my appearance,

CONTINUED ON NEXT PAGE

of weight gain is commonly seen in cultural non-Western societies that feature less pressure to be thin. Even in the United States, Dr. Thomas has worked with many patients who attribute their restrictive eating patterns to uncomfortable feelings of overfullness or a strong need to feel "in control" or "self-disciplined" rather than concerns over shape and weight. Regardless of the rationale for almost anorexic behaviors, their allure can often be difficult to resist.

I have noticed that my view can also shift. But even when it does, my day isn't ruined—or even negatively impacted; I don't love my body any less. I do my best to look at subtle changes in perspective with curiosity rather than fear. For instance, a colleague invited me, on a few occasions recently, to go with her to get our eyebrows waxed. Although I had never considered waxing my eyebrows, her multiple invitations led me to wonder, "Is my facial hair out of control or something?" I remember gazing in the mirror studying what may or may not have been a stray hair above each eye. The difference between now and then is that I quickly recognized what was going on. Instead of continuing with the eyebrow analysis, I just got curious: *Isn't it interesting that I never once thought there was anything wrong with my eyebrows until now?* And the next time my colleague invited me to the salon? I was honest about preferring to connect with her over coffee at our favorite local shop—rather than wincing in pain as our hair got ripped out!

Part 2

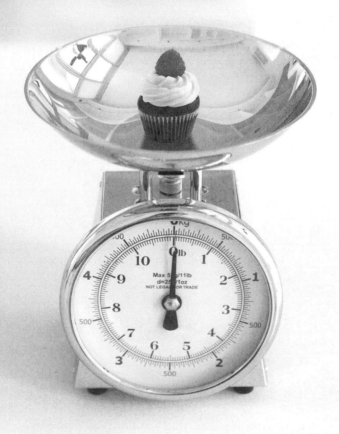

Kicking Ed to the Curb

6

Resisting the Allure of Almost Anorexia

Anorexia's allure is powerful. If you struggle with disordered eating, deciding to change might be the hardest thing you ever do. Many mental illnesses elicit empathy. But anorexia nervosa —the most life threatening of all—is more often met with envy ("You look so thin!") or doubt ("Why can't you just eat?"). If you constantly receive compliments for your restrictive eating behaviors (whether online or face to face), it's easy to think, *I don't have a problem. I'm just healthy.* Then when other people suggest that you seek help, it could be hard to understand why they are so concerned. Although people don't choose to develop almost anorexia, they can certainly choose to be honest with themselves about its real costs and benefits. Those who do are much more likely to make the difficult decision to change.

Wannarexia

Our cultural fascination with self-starvation is not new. According to social historian Joan Jacobs Brumberg, author of

Fasting Girls,[1] medieval saints were revered for their ability to subsist on communion wafers alone. Some—like Catherine of Siena—ultimately starved themselves to death. Later, Victorian "fasting girls" became another miraculous example of the body's alleged ability to live without water or food. But famous faster Sarah Jacob died of malnutrition when physicians used round-the-clock supervision to test her ascetic claims. More recently, so-called breatharians have purported to live on nothing but air. So it was quite a scandal when Wiley Brooks, founder of the Breatharian Institute of America, was caught leaving a convenience store with a hot dog, a Slurpee, and a box of Twinkies.[2] Apparently, he takes his deep breaths with a side of fries.

It's only natural to be intrigued by people who claim to live a food-free lifestyle. After all—as we have learned from the saints, fasting girls, and breatharians—it's not humanly possible. The contemporary admiration of individuals with anorexia nervosa takes this phenomenon a step further. Even though anorexia is now recognized as a deadly mental illness, some still view it in a positive light. Remember that young college student who told Jenni that she wished she had "just a touch of anorexia"? The media has even coined the term *wannarexia* (yes, another –rexia!) to describe individuals who want to become anorexic.[3] Dr. Thomas has seen this phenomenon time and again in her clinical practice. Before becoming acutely ill, many of her patients have ravenously consumed books, movies, and blogs about anorexia, treating them as how-to manuals for developing an eating disorder. Those who stop short at almost anorexia despite these valiant attempts often feel as if they have failed.

If you have never felt this way, it might sound a bit crazy.

Why would anyone want to become anorexic? Well, as individuals with eating disorders know, there are a lot of *perceived* benefits to restricting, bingeing, and purging. In-depth interviews with patients who have eating disorders have identified many apparent pros, such as feeling unique or special, being in control, numbing out emotions, and communicating distress.[4] For those with almost anorexia, these elusive benefits may

---

Jenni's Journey

When I was the thinnest woman in the room, Ed said, "You are special." This became a large part of my identity. If I was stressed out with work or school, Ed gave me permission to "take a break" and binge. I depended on this outlet. When restricting food then numbed the post-binge sadness and frustration, it felt like Ed was lending yet another helping hand. But, as time passed, the behaviors that once provided comfort stopped "working" so well. The high that I had felt from restricting eventually faded—turning into a gnawing anxiety—as my body weakened. And bingeing no longer relieved stress like it had in the past but instead left me feeling even more worried. This is when I realized that I *really* needed to change. Not doing so was killing me mentally, emotionally, physically, and spiritually. Still, in fear, I wondered *Who am I without Ed?* It took some time, but I finally know and learn more each day. I am someone who manages stress without turning to food. I feel my emotions rather than stuffing or starving them. Sometimes these feelings, quite honestly, feel just plain bad. But experiencing difficult emotions has opened the door to some truly amazing ones! Above all, unlike what Ed said, I have learned that, like you, I am special by just being me. None of us is perfect, but rather we are perfectly imperfect—in our own unique ways.

---

feel like a carrot dangling at arm's length, compelling them to continue striving for a full-blown diagnosis that seems just out of reach.

Inspiration or "Thinspiration"?

Triggers to engage in almost anorexic behaviors are everywhere—especially online. An innocent web search on eating disorders could take you directly to a pro-anorexia site. These sites use text, photos, and videos to encourage people to engage in disordered-eating behaviors. Many contain so-called *thinspiration* (thinspo, for short) galleries of emaciated models and celebrities accompanied by dieting slogans. Most contain tips and tricks for restricting, purging, and exercising. The sad truth is that the attitudes and behaviors promoted on these sites are dangerous and, as we discussed in chapter 2, could even be fatal.

Although the mid-2000s saw a public outcry that shut down many pro–eating disorder sites, as of this writing, thinspo material has migrated to new corners of cyberspace—most notably social media platforms like Tumblr,[5] Twitter, and Pinterest. Perhaps more insidiously, thinspo has maintained traction on mainstream sites by donning a thin veneer of social acceptability. Called *fitspiration* (fitspo for short), these new sites claim to motivate people to stay fit. This might sound healthy, yet mantras such as *Skinny girls look good in clothes but fit girls look good naked* have led some to conclude that fitspo may be nothing more than "thinspo in a sports bra."[6] Arguably, fitspo sites promote an even more unattainable body ideal. Now it's not enough to be ultrathin—you have to be ultramuscular too.

Both thinspo and fitspo sites do one thing very well: make people feel bad about themselves. In one experimental study, female college students who viewed a pro-anorexia site felt fatter and more depressed, and reported lower social self-esteem, compared to those who viewed a generic website.[7] Similarly, female undergraduates reported greater body dissatisfaction after viewing photos of thin ultrafit models, compared to normal-weight ultrafit models.[8] And if you think that feeling bad about yourself will motivate you to lose weight, think again. There is absolutely no evidence that viewing pro–eating disorder sites causes people to get thin. Often, this strategy proves to be profitable for site owners who might be selling a weight-loss product on the side or for the webmistress who feels bad about herself. If they can knock you down a bit, then you might just buy their product or be the unwitting object of a downward social comparison.

Creators of pro-anorexia websites most often self-identify as having an eating disorder themselves. They proclaim that anorexia is a lifestyle choice, although they are not living fulfilled lives at all. Why would someone choose to live an unfulfilled life? Because they are working from a place of malnutrition in which they cannot think straight or rationally. Alternatively, they may feel so isolated by the eating disorder that they are driven to create online communities to replace the more authentic offline relationships that they lack. Thus, they are not really making the choice—Ed's in charge. If anorexia were simply a lifestyle choice, then the individuals who fall down the rabbit hole of pro-anorexia could simply decide to stop at some point. But they can't.

We encourage you to see through this web of lies and

manipulation. First, realize that many photographs on these sites are digitally enhanced—not real. Remember Roy Cui's long list of perceived flaws to correct on any image. And professional retouchers aren't the only ones who know how to alter photographs. With today's technology, many people can digitally enhance pictures from home and post them online. Do your best not only to click onto another website but also to talk with a trusted person in your life about any desire you might have to continue viewing material that promotes eating disorders. You can ask another person to help you mediate cyberspace—that is, as long as the individual you choose for support isn't pro-ana. There are plenty of self-love and even anti-thinspiration pages out there. You might decide to start your own positive website, social media site, or blog. The only way to completely avoid tumbling onto fitspo or thinspo is to stay offline. We realize that some people might choose to actively search for these sites after learning about them here or somewhere else. And that is exactly what this chapter is all about—the allure of almost anorexia. If you feel a particular urge to explore one of these harmful sites, the impulse itself may signal that the time to make a healthy change is now.

Personal Recovery Stories

Even recovery-oriented material can sensationalize eating disorders, which is why we have been careful not to add triggering details to the cases presented in this book. Given how many of Dr. Thomas's patients have reported learning tips and tricks from television programs, documentaries, and memoirs, one of her research interests has been the potential for personal recovery stories to glamorize and promote disordered-eating attitudes and behaviors. In one study, she and her colleagues asked middle and high school students to view a brief video on eating disorders in which an attractive female presenter was identified either as someone recovered from an eating disorder or as a health care professional. After viewing the video, girls who watched the video featuring the recovered patient significantly increased their endorsement of statements like "Girls with eating disorders are usually very pretty" and "Girls with eating disorders are especially in control of their lives," while girls who watched the video featuring the health care professional did not increase their endorsement of the same items.[9] In another study, Dr. Thomas randomly assigned female college students to read a graphic anorexia memoir (*Wasted* by Marya Hornbacher) or a control memoir about a young woman with no eating disorder. Although reading the eating disorder memoir did not affect readers' own level of disordered eating compared to the comparison group,[10] participants were more likely to recall positive aspects (such as compliments and pride about dramatic weight loss) than negative aspects (such as health or interpersonal problems) of the author's eating disorder.[11] These empirical data suggest that even well-intentioned recovery-oriented material can convey unintended implicit messages about the benefits of disordered eating. This is why, with her talks and books, Jenni makes a point not to glamorize disordered eating on any level. If you ever hear her speak about her recovery journey, you will notice that the amount of time she tells her "eating disorder story" is quite limited. Rather, she focuses on her "getting better story" and how she tries to live fully today—in a world where Societal Ed reigns and in a body that still has the same personality traits that may have contributed to her becoming ill in the first place.

News outlets may further glamorize anorexia and bulimia by focusing primarily on celebrity cases. In a review of 210 news articles about eating disorders published between 2004 and 2005, 48 percent appeared in the arts and entertainment section, but only 13 percent appeared in health. According to the study investigators, "Newspaper writers are more attuned

Jenni's Journey

"Why didn't you think of that, Jenni?" Ed questioned as I read a memoir that provided specific details about the author's eating disorder. I had picked up the book to gain hope but walked away with a new—and very dangerous—behavior. When I was struggling, it became important for me to realize that Ed read every book alongside me. He also attended my support groups and other recovery appointments. While I worked hard to get better, Ed strategized about how to *never* let that happen. That's the bad news. The good news is that I didn't have to change Ed or his tactics. What I did have to do is change how I responded to him. If Ed urged me to try a destructive tip or trick that he gained from a group or some website, I learned to say no and to take steps toward health instead. Sometimes in response to Ed, I simply said, "Thanks for sharing. But no thanks." I learned that this kind of sarcasm, when used appropriately, could be a powerful recovery tool! If you think about it, Ed is rather boring, always repeating and rephrasing similar ideas over and over again. So, in later recovery, my response to him was often just, "Whatever, Ed," sometimes followed by, "Do you ever have anything new to say?" Yes, a bit more sarcasm. Ed could talk all day long about what he thought I should do, but none of that mattered if I ignored him and chose recovery. What is Ed saying to you right now about this book? More importantly, what do you think?

to [eating disorders] as a source of titillation—a soft topic that belongs on the gossip page along with celebrity divorces and other scandals—than as an issue that deserves serious consideration and possibly societal response."[12] Indeed, all too often, news stories include before (emaciated) and after (healthy) photos, images of the celebrity eating a high-caloric item, and a description of a speedy recovery following a short stint in a spa-like facility. The underlying message seems to be that eating disorders are all about food and weight, and the disorders can be cured rather quickly. Although full healing is absolutely possible, it takes longer than a few weeks to fix something that may have developed over the course of many years. Just because a celebrity can pose for a photo with an ice-cream cone does not mean that he or she is fully recovered.

Taken together, the results of these experimental studies and media analyses suggest that if you (or a loved one) are struggling with almost anorexia, you should watch out for any pro–eating disorder messages you might be receiving, even from seemingly benign sources. If you feel yourself being triggered, shut the anorexia recovery book (even this one!) or switch off the made-for-television movie on bulimia. Pronto.

Blakely

Blakely stealthily cleared the history on her Web browser. She obviously didn't want her parents to find out that she had been visiting a pro-anorexia site. They had reacted dramatically enough when they'd found the lesbian youth association page saved under her "favorites." They still asked her periodically if she'd changed her mind and might be straight. *Ugh. As if.*

Tonight Blakely stumbled upon her favorite pro–eating disorder site yet. After skimming its particularly harsh "warning to wannabes," she clicked her mouse to confirm that she was over eighteen (*Ha—not for three years*) and that she understood the possible health risks associated with eating disorders (*Whatever they are, I'm sure they're a small price to pay for getting thin*). The site finally loaded to reveal the glorious collarbones of Hollywood actress Mary-Kate Olsen and the lithe legs of the nine-girl Korean pop group named Girls' Generation. Even though both Olsen and Girls' Generation had been criticized in the media for being too thin, Blakely thought that they looked amazing. Enthralled, she spent nearly an hour poring over the BMI calculator, calorie counter, and thinspiration gallery.

But the best part, hands down, was meeting her online idol, skinnylove737. Blakely had seen Skinny's posts on other sites; she lived in the same rural state and was the queen of sassy one-liners. Blakely's favorite was, "Broccoli might get stuck in your teeth, but French fries get stuck on your thighs." Apparently, Skinny loved broccoli so much that she even had a floret tattooed to her ankle. (Or at least her profile said so.) With palms sweating, Blakely messaged Skinny through the site's live chat feature:

> perfectc0ntrol: Hey Skinny!
>
> skinnylove737: hey. who's this?
>
> perfectc0ntrol: I'm pro-ana and I really like your posts.
>
> skinnylove737: cool
>
> perfectc0ntrol: What are you eating these days?
>
> skinnylove737: it would probably just be triggering
> if i told you.

> perfectc0ntrol: No it wouldn't. Promise!
>
> skinnylove737: ok. i'm just about to start a 10-day fast. want to join?
>
> perfectc0ntrol: OMG YESS!!!
>
> skinnylove737: cool. let's check in tomorrow.

Snapping her laptop shut, Blakely felt a rush of anticipation. Not only was she starting her first fast; she was doing it in solidarity with Skinny. Even though Blakely didn't have many friends at her new high school, chatting with Skinny gave her an immediate sense of belonging. The next day, Blakely walked the stranger-filled halls with a secret smile, her backpack brimming with calorie-free drinks. When she caught herself looking longingly at the cafeteria's cheeseburgers during lunch period, she pinched her stomach to remind herself of her goal. That night, Skinny cheered her on again via live chat.

But by day 2, Blakely's euphoria gave way to irritation. She couldn't concentrate in trigonometry; all of the numbers reminded her of goal weights and calorie counts. She was starting to feel dizzy and cold. When she got home from school, the scent of her mom's warm apple pie finally pushed her over the edge. She hadn't eaten in one and a half days, and she had to admit she was ravenous. Desperately, she slipped a forkful of forbidden pie into her mouth. After finishing two thick slices, her pangs of hunger became pangs of guilt. *Ugh. How does Skinny do it?*

> perfectc0ntrol: I am so weak.
>
> skinnylove737: what happened?
>
> perfectc0ntrol: Attacked by an apple pie. :(
>
> skinnylove737: you'll do better next time.

perfectc0ntrol: What about you?

skinnylove737: going strong. already losing weight. :)

Blakely was crushed. *I am such a failure*, she thought. Although she was too humiliated to chat with Skinny again, Blakely continued to lurk religiously on the site. Each time Skinny posted about her triumphs in restricting or weight loss, Blakely felt even more worthless. Although she'd lost some weight, it was nowhere near enough to qualify her as "anorexic." She tried a few of the site's purging tips, but she couldn't throw up, no matter how hard she tried. And without even Skinny to talk to, she began to feel increasingly alone. When her mom noticed the site in her smartphone history and insisted she attend a local eating disorder therapy group, Blakely secretly felt relieved. *Maybe someone there will understand me*, she thought.

At the first meeting, the therapist asked each group member to introduce herself and share what had brought her to the group. Blakely was nervous but quickly mumbled her name and a brief description of the smartphone incident. She looked down at the floor shyly during the remaining girls' introductions—but involuntarily snapped to attention when the last girl started speaking.

"When I'm online, I usually talk about how amazing my anorexia is. I mean, I'm still totally pro-ana," the girl said. "But my doctor says that I'm really hurting my body, and inside, I sometimes feel like a fat failure," she whispered, teary-eyed. Blakely felt a chill run down her spine as the girl continued, "A few months ago, I told my fasting buddy that I hadn't eaten anything for days." Blakely's eyes darted downward to the bottom of the girl's capris. There it was—the broccoli tattoo. "The truth is that I only lasted for a few hours before I broke down. I just couldn't stop bingeing and purging."

Blakely knew it. She was positive. It was Skinny.

From the Hair on Your Head to the Tips of Your Toes

Blakely, who was just dabbling in disordered-eating behaviors, had almost anorexia. Before she got professional help, she was well on her way to developing a life-threatening mental illness. What Blakely had originally admired about Skinny turned out to be just an illusion. Skinny wasn't in control of food. Her eating disorder was running the show. And what neither girl realized was that, even if she could hide her identity behind a computer screen, her body couldn't hide from the physical ravages of almost anorexia.

In 1987, the Partnership for a Drug-Free America released what *TV Guide* later named one of the most influential commercials of all time. It showed a man holding up an egg and saying, "This is your brain." After cracking the egg into a frying pan and watching it sizzle, he said, "This is your brain on drugs." After a dramatic pause, he asked, "Any questions?" Although this commercial was specifically referring to narcotics, it could just as easily have applied to almost anorexia. Disordered eating affects nearly every part of your body—from the hair on your head to the tips of your toes.

Physical Changes

You might not care specifically about your hair (which could fall out) or your toes (which may turn blue from poor circulation), but you probably value some of the organs in between.

Let's start with your brain. Blakely noticed that, as her eating disorder progressed, her ability to focus on schoolwork declined. A large number of structural brain imaging studies suggest that, compared to healthy controls, individuals with anorexia show decreased gray matter volume.[13] Gray matter volume is strongly associated with intelligence.[14] So it's no wonder that many individuals with disordered eating report difficulty thinking clearly while underweight. Fortunately, in most studies, brain volume deficits resolve with weight restoration.

Moving downward from the brain, even subclinical levels of disordered eating can have extremely harmful effects. As Jenni knows all too well, being underweight increases your risk for osteoporosis, regardless of the specific eating disorder diagnosis. Furthermore, in a study of 811 female adolescents with EDNOS in a pediatric medical practice, 62 percent met criteria for medical hospitalization (as defined by the American Psychiatric Association and Society for Adolescent Medicine). Specifically, 40 percent were orthostatic by heart rate (you might recognize this in yourself as a "head rush" or dizzy spell). Moreover, 23 percent had bradycardia (low heart rate), 11 percent had severe malnutrition, 4 percent had hypophosphatemia (an electrolyte imbalance that can cause muscle weakness), 3 percent had hypokalemia (an electrolyte imbalance that causes muscle cramping, abnormal heart rhythm, or paralysis), and 3 percent had hypothermia (low body temperature).[15] You don't have to be malnourished or underweight to experience medical complications from almost anorexia, which can also present among those who are overweight or binge eat. In a five-year longitudinal study, individuals with binge eating disorder were significantly more likely than healthy controls to develop components of metabolic syndrome—such as high cholesterol, high blood pressure, and type 2 diabetes—even when known risk factors such as age, sex, and BMI were held constant.[16]

According to Ovidio Bermudez, a physician who specializes in treating the medical complications of eating disorders, "I have had many parents respond with a sigh of relief when I have told them that their loved one 'does not quite fit the diagnostic criteria of anorexia nervosa or bulimia nervosa and thus has EDNOS.' It is not a lesser diagnosis. EDNOS is an eating disorder with different and more often than not just as concerning characteristics and carrying the same risk for medical and psychiatric complications as anorexia or bulimia."[17]

Psychological Changes

Almost anorexia affects individuals psychologically as well as physically. People with eating disorders report many negative cognitive and emotional effects, such as constantly feeling preoccupied with food, disgusted with themselves, guilty or ashamed, less close to others, and like a failure.[18] Interestingly, available data suggest that many of these consequences are due, not to the eating disorder per se, but rather to the well-known effects of malnutrition. In the 1944 Minnesota starvation experiment, thirty-six initially healthy males were asked to cut their food intake in half in order to reach 75 percent of their original body weight. Strikingly, the men experienced many of the psychological symptoms typically seen in individuals with eating disorders, including intense preoccupation with food, ritualistic eating behaviors, mood swings, binge eating, and feelings of fatness.[19] Indeed, longitudinal outcome studies of eating disorders suggest that food restriction is simply not psychologically sustainable in the long term. At least half of individuals with an initial diagnosis of the restricting type of anorexia nervosa eventually cross over to either the binge/ purge type of anorexia nervosa or full-fledged bulimia nervosa.[20] So even though Blakely and Skinny blamed themselves for not sticking to the fast, binge eating is often the body's natural response to starvation.

Mortality Risk

As we discussed in chapter 3, almost anorexia can be deadly. Melissa Avrin, whose life was commemorated in the documentary film *Someday Melissa*,[21] died from a heart attack due to complications from an eating disorder. Tragically, Andrea Smeltzer, whose story you read earlier, is not the only life we have lost. In addition to death from physical complications, suicide is common. In one study, 9 percent of restricting anorexia patients and 25 percent of purging anorexia patients had previously attempted suicide, compared to 0 percent of healthy controls.[22] In other words, despite what you see on pro-anorexia sites or read in the entertainment news, eating disorders are not lifestyle choices and they certainly are not fun. Sometimes, they are such torture that individuals actually take their own lives to escape the pain.

Almost Anorexia: Friend or Foe?

The more you buy in to Ed's false promises, the longer you will struggle with almost anorexia. Dr. Thomas's research with clinical psychologist Sherrie Delinsky has shown that the more a patient's beliefs about Ed's perceived benefits decrease during residential treatment, the less disordered the individual's behaviors and attitudes will be upon discharge.[23] In other words, letting go of the "good" parts of almost anorexia may represent your first step toward health.

Clinical psychologist Lucy Serpell has created a useful exercise that will help you better understand the pros and cons of disordered eating in your own life: writing two letters—friend and foe—to almost anorexia.[24] You might want to address these letters to Ed, Ana, or simply Eating Disorder. Do what works for you. In the first letter, address almost anorexia as if it were your friend. Focus on the function that disordered eating has played in your life and any reasons you would be reluctant to give it up. For example, when Jenni was ill, she would have thanked Ed for making her feel special, giving her a handy excuse for any setbacks in her singing career, or being a friend to her when she felt all alone. These were important factors that kept Ed strong.

In the second letter, write to your eating disorder as if it were your enemy. Focus on what Ed has taken from you—both physically and psychologically—and explore any reasons that you might want to get rid of your eating disorder. Be sure to review your "friend" letter and be honest with yourself about any perceived benefits that might be unrealistic or distorted. For example, for every time Ed told you that you were thin and special, there was probably another time when he told you that you were fat and worthless. Be sure to include those inconsistencies in your enemy letter. In writing this letter, Jenni would have expressed her anger at Ed for making her feel like a failure, giving her osteoporosis, and robbing her of a normal college experience.

Something you might realize from writing your friend and foe letters is that the majority of almost anorexia's pros exist in the short-term, whereas the cons develop over time. If you haven't yet experienced many negative consequences related to your disordered eating, count yourself lucky. If you change now, you can protect yourself. With the help of her mom and her group therapist, that's exactly what Blakely did.

You might choose to share these letters, and their resulting insights, with a trusted person or therapist. Or you might decide to destroy the letters in an effort to let go. Again, do what works for you. Here are Blakely's letters to Ed.

Blakely's Friend and Foe Letters to Almost Anorexia

FRIEND LETTER

Dear Ed,

When I started at my new high school, I felt lonely and lost. Thank you for being there for me when no one else was. You brought me a community of online friends, and you showed me a way to feel special and successful. You even made me feel popular when I became friends with Skinny. You simplified my world—one that can seem so confusing at times. With you, all of life's complications just melted away. Only one thing mattered: being thin. When I was worried about being gay, you comforted me by saying that, as long as I stayed small, everything would be okay. I don't know what I'd do without you to help me manage things.

xoxo,

Blakely

FOE LETTER

Dear Ed,

You ruined my sophomore year of high school. You made me look up to Skinny when it turned out she was lying the whole time about how great you are. You said that the pro-ana girls were my friends, when in reality they don't care about me—they don't even care about themselves! You said that you had my best interests at heart, and I believed you at first, but now I don't. I used to love math before you, but I can hardly add 2 plus 2 when you're around. My parents and I can barely talk with one another these days. And I absolutely hate being cold all of the time! You constantly tell me that I'm fat and not a worthwhile person. Well, I'm sick of it. I don't want you in my life anymore.

Get lost,

Blakely

If you find this letter-writing exercise helpful, consider adding journaling to your list of coping skills. Putting your thoughts in writing can be helpful when you are feeling angry or depressed, although you should be sparing with this skill if you tend to ruminate on negative body image or desire to relapse. Jenni recommends that you remember to journal during the good times too—when you are feeling strong in recovery. Then, when you are feeling bad, you can go back to your journal and remind yourself that it is possible to feel good. It's almost like reading a self-help book that you wrote yourself!

Ready, Set, Go

Recovering from eating disorders is a lot like skydiving. To jump out of a perfectly good airplane, you must trust that your parachute will support you on the way down. If you wait to get absolute proof that your parachute will work before jumping, you will stay in that plane forever—or at least until it runs out of fuel. One thing is for sure: disordered eating is going to stop working for you at some point. Don't wait around for a crash landing. We cannot provide irrefutable evidence that life on the other side of almost anorexia will be better. This is the hard part—it is also where the rewards come in. Only when you jump in skydiving can you experience the exhilarating free fall. And a life without Ed is even better than that.

Ready to jump out of that plane—to begin a life free from almost anorexia? The very first step is normalizing your eating.

7

Do the Next Right Thing
Normal Eating

In a world enamored with restricting food—both the amount and the variety—combining the words *normal* and *eating* can be confusing. What is normal anyway? You have probably heard "normal eating" used alongside the names of popular diets, but we assure you that diets are far from normal. On the road to recovery from almost anorexia, we suggest a two-phase approach to normalizing your eating. The first phase focuses on *external* cues. Eating at regular intervals throughout the day (such as breakfast, lunch, dinner, and snacks) and reducing any bingeing and purging are the main goals of this phase. The second phase focuses on *internal* cues—called "intuitive eating." This is a nondiet approach to food first described by dietitians Evelyn Tribole and Elyse Resch in their book of the same name. Broadening your food choices and honoring your true likes and dislikes during this intuitive phase will help you to break the rigid dietary rules that keep you imprisoned.

Phase One: External Cues

As young children, we learn to eat based on external cues. We might wake up for breakfast at 7 a.m., because we have to be ready for the school bus at 8 a.m. We then eat pizza for lunch just because it happens to be what is served in the cafeteria. At the end of the day, we might sit down for a home-cooked dinner and eat what our parents serve. Unfortunately, individuals with almost anorexia have typically lost touch with this once-familiar eating pattern. Instead of eating by the clock, they may eat (or not eat) primarily to manage their shape, weight, or emotions. If you have been bingeing (like Abriana), purging (like Camille), or juice fasting (like Taylor), the first phase of normalizing your eating is to structure it—just like you did as a kid.

When Should I Eat?

A basic structure for eating includes breakfast, lunch, dinner, and a couple of snacks. As a rule of thumb, try not to go more than four hours without food.[1] The optimal timing of eating will depend on your daily schedule. For example, a busy working mom might eat breakfast with her kids at 6 a.m., lunch at work at 11 a.m., a snack at her desk at 3 p.m., and dinner with her family at 6 p.m. and then share a bowl of popcorn with her husband at 8 p.m. after the kids have gone to bed. On the other hand, a college student might sleep late and have breakfast at 10 a.m. before class, lunch at 2 p.m. after class, snack after sports practice at 5 p.m., dinner at the dining hall at 8 p.m., and an evening study snack at 11 p.m. Adhering to her own personalized structure helped Taylor avoid the juice fasting that often triggered her peanut butter binges.

Certain rituals at mealtimes can help you create this pattern. People tend to binge at places other than the kitchen table—possibly at the refrigerator door, in the car, or even on the bathroom floor. So, for many, creating a comfortable place to sit down at the table is important. You might consider lighting a candle or playing music. Say a prayer if you think this might help you to connect with some serenity. When Ed screamed in Jenni's ears at mealtimes, a quick prayer often turned down the volume and—even if just a notch—brought her closer to peace.

Sharing meals with significant others may also help you normalize your eating pattern. In a large-scale study of adolescent girls, eating five or more family meals per week was associated with a reduced risk of developing disordered-eating behaviors five years later.[2] Similarly, leading treatments for anorexia enlist mealtime support from both parents and partners.[3] Knowing that you are accountable to someone who cares about you can make all the difference. In *Brave Girl Eating*, Harriet Brown wrote about refeeding her anorexic daughter, Kitty, who was quite vigilant about whether her parents were watching her at mealtimes. Harriet recalled, "Kitty asks again and again whether we're watching, and I know she's really asking: *You're making me eat this, right? I don't have any choice here. Do I?* She needs us to take the responsibility for her eating because the compulsion not to eat is still so powerful."[4] Not all people who struggle with disordered eating require this intense level of support, but everyone does, in fact, need some support around food. Find what works best for you or your loved one.

What Should I Eat?

If you are reading this book, you probably already spend a lot of time thinking about calories and carbs. Dr. Thomas typically finds that her patients are just as knowledgeable about nutrition as she is (if not more so!). The problem is that they obsess over the details rather than putting broad principles into practice. At the height of her illness, Jenni knew exactly how many fat grams were in a slice of cheese, but she would never let herself add one to a sandwich.

That's why we are not going to tell you *what* to eat. *When* you eat is much more important when you first start out to change your eating. If you are genuinely curious about which foods are healthy for you, we invite you to visit the Harvard School of Public Health's Nutrition Source website (www.hsph .harvard.edu/nutritionsource). Based on the latest scientific research, physician and nutrition researcher Walter Willet and his colleagues have created a healthy eating guide comprising a combination of fruits, vegetables, whole grains, proteins, and oils. But even these are just guidelines. Please don't fall into the trap of replacing one set of rigid rules with another. To help in the food department, consider seeing a registered dietitian who has experience in treating patients who struggle with disordered eating. During her recovery, Jenni found dietary counseling to be invaluable.

When selecting what to eat, try to anticipate how long the meal or snack will satiate you. Clinical psychologist Linda Craighead, author of *The Appetite Awareness Workbook*, has suggested a two-hour rule: "Each time you eat, eat enough so that you are not likely to be biologically hungry for at least two hours." For example, "It is important to understand that one piece of fruit is not an adequate snack. It will not keep you from being hungry for two hours."[5] In other words, try some peanut butter with that banana!

An important caveat with food is that individuals who have been eating very little and/or are extremely underweight are at risk of refeeding syndrome, a potentially fatal complication of increasing energy intake too rapidly. If any of the following apply to you, consult your physician before attempting to normalize your eating:

1. Your BMI is less than 16.0.

2. You have unintentionally lost more than 15 percent of your original body weight in the past three to six months.

3. You have eaten little or nothing in the past ten days.

4. Your recent laboratory results have found low levels of potassium, phosphorus, or magnesium.[6]

Jenni's Journey

"Think back to a time when you had a normal relationship with food," my dietitian encouraged. These words—meant to inspire hope—did quite the opposite, because I couldn't think of such a time. As far back as I could remember, I was disordered around food—at least a little. My friends enjoyed Happy Meals at McDonald's while I hunted for the toy inside, afraid of eating the fattening food. Even though I had no previous experience with "normal," I still had to find it. And my dietitian helped me to do just that. Obviously, in the beginning, the idea of listening to my body sounded like a foreign concept, and I wondered,

CONTINUED ON NEXT PAGE

CONTINUED FROM PREVIOUS PAGE

Can anyone really do that? When I tried to listen, I had the strange feeling that my body was giving me the silent treatment. Other than knowing when I was famished from not eating or overstuffed after bingeing, I didn't hear a thing. To get back in touch, I had to do whatever it took to fuel my body on a regular basis. The difficulty of carrying out this seemingly simple task cannot be overstated. I ultimately came to understand that eating becomes easy by eating—not by simply talking or journaling about it. I also learned that one of my biggest fears—that I might never stop eating (that is, binge constantly) if I began to eat in a more normal way—did not come true. Slowly, over time, I began to notice more subtle cues when I was hungry and when I was full. Today, I can actually distinguish between what types of foods my body wants—from fruits and vegetables to protein and fat or all of the above. I still can't think back to an earlier time when I was normal with food. But I'm grateful to say that I am living it now!

But I Don't Trust My Body Yet

The reason we recommend starting with external cues is that, in early recovery from almost anorexia, you and your body might not trust one another. Maybe you haven't given your body food in a balanced way for so long that it doesn't know—from meal to meal—whether you are going to starve or stuff it. When you do eat, you don't trust what is going to happen. *Will my body's ravenous hunger lead to bingeing? Will my body hold on to every calorie in fear of my never feeding it again?* In other words, according to dietitian Evelyn Tribole, coauthor of *Intuitive Eating*, when you have almost anorexia, your "satiety meter is broken."[7]

At least part of the reason is biological. Disordered eating often leads to delayed gastric emptying. In one study, it took women with anorexia six hours for a standard test meal of pasta with meat sauce to exit their stomachs, whereas it took less than four hours for healthy controls.[8] No wonder that, in another study, 89 percent of patients with almost anorexia and other eating disorders complained of nausea and/or abdominal bloating after eating an ordinary size meal.[9] Jenni remembers this painful sensation all too well. After eating a normal lunch in her early recovery days, it felt like the food was sitting in her stomach *forever*, not moving. Five hours later, when others were hungry for dinner, she still felt completely full, as if she'd just eaten.

But we aren't letting you off the hook. You still have to eat to get better. Gastric emptying time typically speeds up as food intake normalizes. In other words, it takes time, but you can reconnect with your body's signals, including hunger and fullness cues that tell you when to eat and when to stop. You will also begin to get a sense of what types of food your body is craving. Just making an effort to be conscious of your body's signals is a step in the right direction. In the beginning, this might mean that you attempt to pay attention but that you hear absolutely nothing—radio silence. That's okay. Simply paying attention is key.

The Next Right Thing

One of Jenni's favorite sayings is *Do the next right thing*. This has become a motto for many people trying to normalize their eating. Having slipups and setbacks along the way is expected. The important thing to remember is to get back on track as soon as possible. That means right now, not tomorrow.

Doing the next right thing and all-or-nothing thinking cannot coexist. Remember Abriana? If she ate just one morsel of food beyond her "diet plan," she thought she had blown it, so she just went ahead and binged for the rest of the day. Telling yourself that you've already "messed up" and therefore have permission to "mess up" more will only continue the disordered-eating cycle. It won't help keep you on track. Abriana eventually realized that one "extra" bite of food wouldn't negatively affect her body and that the best strategy for getting fully better from disordered eating was to always eat the very next meal or snack in a balanced way.

In Jenni's experience, the hardest cycle to break was "making up" for a binge. When she binged, Ed would say, in no uncertain terms, that she must make up for it. And as long as Jenni listened, she wasn't getting better. Not making up for a binge by purging or fasting seemed unthinkable. But it wasn't. It was just extraordinarily uncomfortable. Doing the next right thing —not purging and eating the next meal after a binge—meant feeling bad for a while. But in the long run, it is what broke the cycle of disordered eating and what led to feeling good. No, make that feeling great.

Trying to restrict your food to "make up" for a binge might sound like a good idea at the time, but research suggests it only perpetuates the binge-diet cycle. In one study, women with bulimia nervosa were asked to record when they binged and the extent to which they restricted their calorie intake each day during a two-week period. The more they restricted, the more likely they were to binge that same day, and even the next day—twenty-four hours later.[10] Just telling yourself you are going on a diet tomorrow can cause you to overeat tonight; this is a phenomenon psychologists call the "last supper effect." In one study, chronic dieters ate more cookies in a fake taste test when they were assigned to start a reduced-calorie diet immediately afterward than those who were not being asked to go on a diet.[11]

Stop Stuffing and Starving Emotions

Normal eating means that from time to time you eat just because you are happy, often wanting to share the moment with someone else. At Dr. Thomas's *Breakfast at Tiffany's* themed bridal shower, her best friends Emily and JennyBess baked her a platter of cupcakes designed to look like gift boxes from Tiffany and Co., with pale blue frosting and little white bows. Even though she wasn't especially hungry, she still ate two! Normal eating also means that you might eat for comfort sometimes when you are sad or lonely. But the key words in those last couple of sentences are "from time to time" and "sometimes." We all eat based on emotions occasionally, but using food to deal with feelings on a regular basis lies at the heart of almost anorexia.

Food is fuel, not a coping mechanism for life. When Jenni's treatment team first told her that she was using her eating disorder, in part, to starve and stuff away feelings, she didn't believe them. Only when she stopped stuffing and starving her body with food did she eventually see and feel the truth. Intense emotions rose to the surface, and in the beginning, it felt awful. Like many people in this phase, Jenni wondered, *Why did I recover just to feel this bad?* But this was, in fact, just a phase—not the end of the journey. Jenni learned other ways to cope with feelings, like calling a friend, writing in her journal, and simply being present. Eventually, she learned to experience the feeling, knowing that if she did, it would eventually pass.

In women with bulimia, negative emotions—such as guilt, fear, and sadness—increase in the four hours leading up to a binge, purge, or binge/purge episode, and decrease in the four hours afterward.[12] In other words, bingeing and purging are powerful emotion-regulation strategies. You wouldn't be doing them if they weren't so effective. To break the cycle, you will need to brainstorm a list of alternative ways to manage difficult feelings. Here are some ideas that Dr. Thomas's patients have found effective:

- spending time with friends
- talking on the phone
- going for a walk
- listening to music
- watching funny television shows

No longer using food to manage your emotions is tough, but Kaitlyn was able to do it.

Kaitlyn

I wonder if my birth parents were like this with food? Kaitlyn wondered, as she carefully counted the number of grapes equaling one serving and placed them one by one into a sandwich bag for lunch. While she deeply loved her parents who had adopted her from Korea at birth, their carefree and relaxed attitude toward food had always been just one more reminder that she didn't quite fit in—anywhere. Years out of high school, at age thirty-three, Kaitlyn still lived much of her life as if she were still within those locker-lined halls. Growing up in

America with a white family who didn't know much about her cultural background, she had always felt different from the other Asian kids. And she could never let go of the fact that she didn't look like the white kids. Dreading the lunchroom where the tables always seemed to divide by ethnicity, Kaitlyn would just join whoever invited her to sit down first. And since she was well liked by all with her bubbly personality (to hide her underlying insecurities), that usually didn't take long.

On her way out the door of her chic studio apartment, Kaitlyn stopped to make sure that she had placed the right number of turkey slices on her sandwich when her smartphone buzzed with a reminder: "First therapy appointment today!" Grabbing a notebook, she thought, *Hopefully, I will finally get some answers.* Kaitlyn had decided to talk with a therapist at the local center that treated obsessive-compulsive disorder. Following work that day at the marketing firm where she was a lead consultant, she headed to the appointment both excited and anxious to see what therapy was all about.

"I can't stop thinking about food," she told the therapist. "After seeing a website a few years ago that lists exact serving sizes for every food imaginable, the numbers just won't leave my head." Quickly realizing that Kaitlyn's obsessions centered around food and weight, the therapist referred her to outpatient eating disorder treatment with Dr. Thomas. *But I don't have a problem with eating,* Kaitlyn thought.

She was right. From one perspective, she didn't technically have a problem with eating. Kaitlyn ate enough calories every day to sustain a healthy body. Although thin, she was never too thin. But her body was a point of confusion for her and always had been. Although her white friends had always complimented her figure, she never felt quite thin enough to be Asian. Kaitlyn wasn't sure what size she was supposed to be, but she did know one thing: she would never gain weight. She still prided herself for being able to fit into her high school prom dress.

Even though Kaitlyn ate enough and rarely missed a meal, her attitude with food was so rigid that it was disrupting her life. When she dined with clients at regular work dinners, she often panicked upon the food's arrival: *How many servings is this? Should I put half in a to-go box now or later?* Normally, Kaitlyn was good at putting her clients at ease, but they became noticeably uncomfortable around the dinner table. And Kaitlyn's dating life was nonexistent. Because she had to eat at restaurants so much for work, she just couldn't bear the thought of dining out yet again during the week. She hated that guys always asked her out to share a meal. *Why does everything seem to revolve around food?* Constant thoughts of calories and planning the perfect meals absorbed most of her time.

In therapy with Dr. Thomas, Kaitlyn kept saying, "But I eat." She didn't understand why she was in an eating disorder clinic. Dr. Thomas helped her to realize that although her caloric intake was adequate, she needed to work on her disordered attitude toward food. She needed to add flexibility, not calories. This, in part, landed Kaitlyn in the category of unspecified feeding and eating disorders. Breaking food rules would be a big part of Kaitlyn's recovery. In the beginning, Kaitlyn couldn't imagine eating, for instance, even just one grape over the recommended serving size. If she took a banana out of the fruit bowl at work, she always tried to take the smallest one. Eating a tiny amount over what she was "supposed to" created such feelings of intense shame and guilt that she sometimes would refer to these instances as a binge. And these "binges" inevitably led to body loathing. It was as if she could pinpoint exactly on her body where each "extra" morsel of food was appearing.

To help improve Kaitlyn's attitude with food, Dr. Thomas recommended many strategies. Kaitlyn began connecting more with trusted friends at mealtimes. Watching how and what they ate—an external cue—she realized that no one eats "perfectly." She also experimented with trying new recipes and saw first-hand that exact measurements didn't matter that much. (You'll read later how Kaitlyn stood up to a bunch of grapes.) Slowly, she began to trust her body more, understanding that it could make up for small differences in amounts eaten. Unlike what Kaitlyn originally expected from therapy, Dr. Thomas also encouraged her to broaden her sense of self-worth. At first, she didn't even know what that meant and had no idea where to start. But then, at Dr. Thomas's suggestion, she began volunteering at a local children's hospital. The kids' genuine excitement about seeing her each week helped to melt some feelings of not being good enough, as did changing up her dating routine. She joined an online dating site and challenged herself to go out on at least one date every few weeks. One of her favorite dates was going to the ice-cream parlor with Kevin where they shared a magnificent sundae—calories and serving size unknown.

Kaitlyn got better over a period of six months. Through the process, she learned how almost anorexia had been, in part, a way for her to cope with always feeling "different." So healing meant that she finally started to feel good enough—just as she was. The amount of food she ate stayed about the same. Her weight remained steady. What changed was her attitude toward it all.

Phase Two: Internal Cues

Moving from relying on external cues to internal cues is the next step in achieving normal eating. Research suggests that the three core features of intuitive eating include (1) eating for physical (rather than emotional) reasons, (2) relying on internal hunger and satiety cues, and (3) giving yourself unconditional permission to eat.[13] Put more simply, according to Tribole and Resch, "Intuitive eaters march to their inner hunger signals, and eat whatever they choose without experiencing guilt or an ethical dilemma."[14] When Kaitlyn first started therapy, she was the opposite of an intuitive eater. She ate to give herself a sense of control—not because she was hungry. In fact, she was terrified to even admit when she felt hungry, craved a food that was not on her "OK list," or wanted even one morsel more than the serving size indicated on the package label. Through treatment, she discovered that food is just food, connected with her hunger and satiety cues, and came to recognize all of her damaging food rules—and broke them. In time, you can too.

Food Is Just Food

Have you ever noticed the labels and names that we give to certain foods? Light, low-calorie vanilla sponge cake is called "angel food," whereas buttery, rich chocolate cake is referred to as "devil's food." The names alone imply that food has a moral value: good versus bad. But if you choose high-calorie devil's food cake over the angelic variety, you are not bad. Food doesn't have a moral value. It is just food. Of course, it's hard to remember this in real life. In one study, women—both with and without eating disorders—felt guiltier and fatter after merely being asked to *imagine* eating a high-calorie food.[15]

Think about a recent time you dined out with others. While looking at the menu, you might have heard someone say something like, "I've been good all day. Now, I'm going to be bad." And this person isn't talking about dining and dashing but rather ordering the decadent cheesecake. Although stealing the cheesecake might be considered morally wrong, simply eating it isn't. Begin to notice this kind of dialogue within your own mind and those around you. If your loved one is struggling with almost anorexia, do your best to minimize negative food talk, which enforces the allure of anorexia. Most people want to be "good," and Ed says that you are good if you restrict calories. In fact, with anorexia, you reach the highest point of goodness according to the senseless morality of food rules.

Do you categorize foods into good and bad? If so, you might have noticed that the bad list has grown longer and longer over time, possibly leaving only a few good items that you can eat with impunity. But all food has its place in normal eating. Even though a bowl of berries might be packed with more nutrients than a chocolate-chip cookie, that doesn't mean that cookies are bad and that you should never eat them.

Your body needs different foods at various times. Ed Tyson, a physician who specializes in eating disorders, told us that he explains it to patients this way: "Imagine a scenario where you are driving down a road in Darfur, Africa. You come up on someone who is starving and you have two choices to feed them something: (1) a Greek salad with some feta cheese, julienned vegetables, and dressing, or (2) a Big Mac with double meat, double cheese, fries, and a shake. Which choice has the most of what this starving person needs, i.e., which is the healthier choice for this person? The one with the most calories, protein, and fat is what would give a starving person more of what they need—the Big Mac choice. So, what is 'healthy' is really relative and is dependent on the needs of the individual at that time."[16] We aren't saying that everyone's road to recovery must include a McDonald's drive-through, but if you are currently underweight, increasing the energy density of your diet is critical to healing.

Intuitive Eating

All of this "listen to your body" stuff may sound like a bunch of mumbo-jumbo. But you may have noticed by now that Dr. Thomas is pretty obsessed with science. There is actually very good research to suggest that intuitive eating interventions (that is, those designed to enhance appetite awareness and encourage eating in response to physical hunger cues) are effective in reducing eating disorder symptoms.[17] To put intuitive eating into practice, check out the phase 2 column of table 6. Important to note: you might see yourself on both sides of the table—in phase 1 and phase 2—on any given day. That's okay. What matters is that your general progression is to the right— toward internal cues.

Intuitive drinking is also important. No, we are not talking about cocktails, but rather actual fluid consumption. Although there is controversy surrounding how much water you really need (the often-cited eight glasses a day is not scientifically based), most health care professionals agree that you should drink to your thirst. Unfortunately, many people with almost anorexia and other officially recognized eating disorders do not. In one study, 25 percent reported drinking too little (to punish themselves or feel in control), whereas 63 percent were drinking too much (in an attempt to suppress appetite or

Table 6.

Normal Eating Means . . .

Phase One: External Cues	Phase Two: Internal Cues
1. You work hard not to engage in eating-disordered behaviors like restricting, bingeing, or purging.	1. Eating-disordered behaviors don't really come to mind. They aren't an option. It's easy.
2. You eat at regular intervals, not going for more than four hours without eating. You don't allow yourself to get too hungry, which could lead to bingeing. Sometimes, you might even feel as if you eat like a robot.	2. You eat based on internal rather than external cues, noticing subtle feelings of hunger rather than waiting to eat until you are famished and stopping only when you are completely stuffed. Yet, you are flexible.
3. Food is fuel. You do your best not to view food as "good" or "bad," but even if you do, you eat it anyway.	3. Food is neutral. Certain items are not labeled as "good" or "bad," and there is nothing you forbid yourself to eat.
4. You notice Ed's food rules in your life and begin to challenge them.	4. You no longer base when and how much you eat on Ed's rules.
5. With planning and support, you challenge yourself to try new foods and new eating situations (such as birthday cake or dining out).	5. You spontaneously try new foods and diverse eating experiences. Dining out with others and attending social events is enjoyable.
6. You eat according to guidelines and structure—usually three meals a day with two or three snacks.	6. You eat according to your body's needs, creating a flexible structure that helps you stay strong and healthy. You eat what you want and when you crave it—in balance.
7. If you are not in the mood for food, but you know that you need to eat in order to support your recovery, you do it anyway.	7. If you are not in the mood for a particular type of food, you don't force yourself to eat it. Instead, you choose something that sounds satisfying to you.
8. You pay attention to relevant health information, focusing on adding healthy foods you may be missing in your diet.	8. You pay some attention to nutrition and take into account your relevant health information, but you don't let this become rigid and interfere with balanced eating.
9. You purposefully practice healthy self-soothing skills instead of using food to manage your emotions.	9. Eating is enjoyable but is not used as a coping mechanism for negative emotions.
10. You don't feel comfortable "going off" your structured plan.	10. You occasionally eat a little more or less than usual in response to social factors or proximity to food, and you don't beat yourself up about this.

This table can be downloaded at www.almostanorexic.com.

facilitate purging).[18] With regard to alcohol and other drugs, women with either an eating or substance use disorder are four times more likely to develop the other disorder compared to women with neither problem.)[19] Misuse of alcohol and other drugs might reduce your distress in the moment, but in the long run it will only make you feel worse and will likely exacerbate your disordered eating. If you think substance abuse might be a problem for you and you can't control your drinking or drug use on your own, we recommend getting help.

When "Normal" Doesn't Feel So Normal

Right now, disordered eating might be the norm for you or your loved one. Without question, people with almost anorexia are signing up to feel quite abnormal when they first try to eat normally. In this way, feeling weird, bad, or just completely unbalanced is actually a step in the right direction.

People who struggle with disordered eating adhere to certain "food rules" that give them a false sense of security and control. Dividing items into good and bad categories is just one type of food rule, but many others exist. For example, *I absolutely cannot eat between meals. Dessert is allowed only once per week.* These rules, of course, don't truly provide safety, because they inevitably lead to being out of control with food and feeling miserable. When Dr. Thomas talks with patients about their own individual food rules in group therapy, these patients' rules feel normal to them. While someone might say that Ed never allows her to eat ice cream, another might share that Ed forces him to binge on gallons of ice cream. One woman might say that Ana lets her eat whatever she wants in the morning but requires intense restriction during the rest of the day, and a man sitting next to her might have an Ed who enforces the opposite rule. If all of these food rules were followed, you would not be allowed to eat anything at all or, on the flip side, you would have to eat everything all of the time. Some rules really are meant to be broken.

Breaking the Rules

Most people don't like being told what to do, yet many let Ed boss them around. Chapter 4 included an exercise asking you to identify your dietary rules. You may have noticed that you are avoiding certain foods, eating only at specific times, or restricting the overall amount that you eat—all because Ed promises you that following these rules will keep you thin, safe, binge-free, or something else. In this exercise, we'd like you to get curious about whether these rules are truly serving you.

Specifically, we invite you to design an experiment. Behavioral experiments are a helpful strategy in the treatment of eating disorders, including almost anorexia.[20] Before diving in, take a look at Kaitlyn's example in table 7. Also, consider talking about this exercise with someone you trust, like a therapist, dietitian, or supportive friend or family member. Following the steps listed in table 8, we encourage you to identify one of your dietary rules and think about what Ed has told you will happen if you break that rule. (Use table 8 or a notebook. You can also download this exercise at www.almostanorexic.com.) Because Ed does not always speak in scientific hypotheses (he's not that clever), it may help to ask yourself, *Why am I so afraid to break this rule?* Ed may have told you, for example, "Eating chocolate will make you fat" or "If you eat a normal-size dinner, your feelings of fullness will be so unbearable that you will not possibly be able to cope."

Once you have identified Ed's prediction, try to design a simple experiment to test it. Be scientific. If you eat a bar of chocolate, for example, how will you know whether you have "gotten fat"? Simply *feeling* fatter doesn't count, since these feelings are more strongly correlated with mood than with BMI. Could you try on the same pair of jeans that morning and again the next day? Could you weigh yourself? This is the only time we would actually encourage you to body check. We told you, Dr. Thomas will do anything for science. However, even Dr. Thomas agrees: if weighing yourself will feel unsupportive to your recovery right now, design an experiment that doesn't require any numbers—like Kaitlyn did in table 7. Once you have designed your experiment, consider possible alternative predictions. For example, maybe you will feel fatter (but not weigh more) after eating the chocolate. Maybe nothing at all will happen. Although it's possible that Ed has been telling you the truth all along (maybe you *are* a very special person who really will gain ten pounds from eating just one square of chocolate), chances are he's way off the mark. The only way you'll know for sure is to carry out the experiment. That's how Kaitlyn finally overcame her obsession with weighing and measuring food. In a similar way, this exercise helped Emma realize that she could tolerate the anxiety of eating odd (rather than even) numbers of foods. And remember Camille who was trapped in her macrobiotic diet? She learned from this very exercise that eating "regular" food would not, in fact, make her sick.

Keep challenging yourself. If you create an experiment and receive surprising pro-recovery results that you don't quite believe, do it again. Repeat until you do believe. In Dr. Thomas's research, she's always doing experiments over and over—

Table 7.

Kaitlyn's Behavioral Experiment with Grape Servings

1. Describe a dietary rule you try to follow in order to influence your weight or prevent binge eating.

   Never eat more than <u>exactly</u> one serving of grapes at any given time.

2. What does Ed predict will happen if you break this rule? How would you know if that came true?

   If I break this rule, Ed says that I will eventually lose control of my eating in general. One extra grape will lead to an extra slice of pizza and then to an extra cookie—to eventual out-of-control bingeing. I will know if this prediction comes true if I do, in fact, begin bingeing in the next few days after eating an extra grape.

3. How can you design an "experiment" to test the accuracy of Ed's prediction?

   I will eat one extra grape with each serving (once a day) for a week. At the end of the week, I will let Dr. Thomas know if I have binged or had the desire to.

4. What are possible alternative predictions? Since Ed is great at catastrophizing, he might have some more predictions. Also, are there any possible *positive* outcomes?

   Ed says that I might become so upset after eating more than a serving that I won't be able to function at work. I might lose my job if this continues. Or, maybe, nothing will happen. I might be okay. Maybe I can eat grapes without obsessing!

5. Complete the experiment. What actually happens?

   Eating one extra grape did not cause me to want to binge eat. I feel a little freer knowing that one little grape can't control my life anymore. It feels good.

Table 8.
**Design a Behavioral Experiment to
Test Your Prediction about a Dietary Rule**

1. Describe a dietary rule you try to follow in order to influence your weight or prevent binge eating.
2. What does Ed predict will happen if you break this rule? How would you know if that came true?
3. How can you design an "experiment" to test the accuracy of Ed's prediction?
4. What are possible alternative predictions? Since Ed is great at catastrophizing, he might have some more predictions. Also, are there any possible *positive* outcomes?
5. Complete the experiment. What actually happens?

This table can be downloaded at www.almostanorexic.com.

making sure she got it right the first time. On the other hand, if you design an experiment and your results seem to indicate that Ed has been right all along, think again. Maybe, for instance, you do happen to gain a few pounds one week when you allowed yourself to eat dessert. This doesn't definitively mean that a couple of chocolate-chip cookies led to weight gain. Consider any other variables that might have affected the results: For example, did you change anything else about your eating during the same time period? Are you feeling bloated due to constipation, menstruation, or water retention? And maybe you could take the test even further. How will gaining a couple of pounds truly affect you? Maybe Ed predicts that your life will be over if you gain a few pounds. Ask yourself: Is my life really over? In one way or another, your experiment will teach you an important lesson.

Are You Just Trying to Make Me Fat?

Many individuals recovering from disordered eating believe that books, clinicians, and others are just trying to make them fat. Dr. Thomas's patients are sometimes pretty suspicious when they first start working with her. But we seriously have no interest in making you fat. This isn't *Hansel and Gretel*—where a wicked witch lures children into her candy-decorated house to fatten them up in preparation for eating them. Rather, our goal is to help you function better, mentally as well as physically. And that's a lot more than Ed can say.

You may be wondering how you can eat several times per day—and even enjoy cupcakes—while maintaining a healthy body weight. Here's how: on average, the more you weigh, the more calories your body burns—even while you rest. Researchers can predict your resting metabolic rate with a fairly straightforward equation (such as the Harris-Benedict). Studies suggest, however, that individuals with anorexia burn fewer calories per day (about 200 to 380 fewer, to be exact) than such equations would predict.[21] In other words, while people are starved, their metabolism is artificially suppressed. Healthy people of similar body mass are burning about a cupcake's worth more calories per day simply by not undereating. Fortunately, as people with anorexia are refed, their resting metabolic rate returns to the level of healthy individuals.[22] Dr. Thomas calls this phenomenon the "cupcake catch-up."

If you are currently underweight, you'll need to gain enough weight to reach a healthy level in order to experience this metabolic boost. When it comes down to it, your final body weight will be determined greatly by your genes. We could all eat the exact same amount and exercise in the same way for an entire year and we would all look different. If you are wondering what will happen to your weight when you start eating normally, consider your previous adult weights (if you had previously healthy ones). Research suggests that individuals who are weight suppressed (that is, their current weight is much lower than their highest adult weight) tend to gain slightly more weight during anorexia and bulimia treatment compared to eating disorder patients who are not weight suppressed, but the difference is usually pretty small.[23]

So you'll need to prepare for some suspense. It's completely normal for your weight to fluctuate in early recovery. When Jenni first stopped using compensatory behaviors to "make up for" binges, she gained more weight than she had anticipated. (She was still bingeing a lot.) It took about a year more in recovery for her weight to stabilize. Until then, she believed her treatment team had succeeded in making her fat, which Ed thought was their entire goal! One of Dr. Thomas's patients used to call her crying every time she gained a pound. Now this woman's weight is stable and she takes minor fluctuations in stride.

In the End, Food Is the Best Medicine

You can read this book one hundred times—even memorize it word for word—but if you are not eating, it doesn't matter. Neither does therapy and all of the other best intentions. Food is the best medicine when it comes to recovering from almost anorexia. Without a doubt, you absolutely cannot get better without it. You must find balance with food, a difficult but very possible task. There is no way to make tackling the food easy. As we said before, you must just jump right into the hard part. You will have lapses along the way, but they won't last forever. Despite how long destructive behaviors and attitudes have been entrenched in your life, you can develop a healthy relationship with food.

People often think that they are completely unique, the only person in the world who cannot get better. But we have known many people who thought this, including Kaitlyn and Jenni, who got fully better. You can too. Eventually, normal eating will become your default position, your natural place. And this is possible not only with food but also in other areas of your life, including exercise.

- ◆ -

8

Get Moving (or Not)
What's Best for You?

"Unless you puke, faint, or die, keep walking!" celebrity personal trainer Jillian Michaels exhorted power-walking *Biggest Loser* contestants in the season 6 premiere.¹ The viral spread of this quote, from fitspiration websites to athletic tees, suggests that there may be no such thing as too much exercise in our fitness-obsessed culture. But if you have almost anorexia, it's possible that you are exercising too much, too hard, or for the wrong reasons. Alternatively, if you feel constantly worried that you are too out of shape to wear spandex in public, almost anorexia could be your biggest barrier to breaking a sweat. Intuitive exercise, which we'll introduce in this chapter, means listening to your body (not Ed!) when it comes to movement. Exercise can be hard work, but it should be something you look forward to, not something you dread.

How Much Is Too Much?

When it comes to exercise frequency, everyone has an opinion. Canadian workout-wear company Lululemon Athletica, purveyor of yoga and running gear, says we should "sweat once a day."[2] The U.S. Surgeon General, who does not, to our knowledge, earn income from yoga pant sales, recommends at least "150 minutes of moderate-intensity physical activity per week" (for adults) and "1 hour of daily physical activity" (for children and teenagers).[3] On the other hand, you may have seen warnings about the dangers of compulsive exercise, excessive exercise, overexercise, or even exercise addiction. So how do you know if you are doing too much of a good thing?

After lengthy debates about the number of hours per week that could distinguish "excessive" from "nonexcessive" exercise, eating disorder researchers have concluded that problematic exercise behavior is more about quality than quantity. Specifically, viewing exercise as obligatory, exercising primarily to change weight and shape, and feeling guilty after missing an exercise session are more strongly related to disordered-eating attitudes and behaviors than the actual amount of time spent working out. In other words, exercising compulsively—because you *have* to, not because you *want* to—is a much better marker of almost anorexia or another eating disorder than exercising excessively.[4] Unfortunately, Daniela struggled with both.

Daniela

As a high school senior and incoming captain of her cross-country team, Daniela was born to run. Ever since she was little, she loved to feel the dirt on her heels and the wind in her face. Nearly every summer evening, she slipped on her sneakers, looped a house key through her shoelace, and chased after a "runner's high" along the beach. Sometimes her little brother Alberto tagged along. She always slowed down to match his little-kid pace and sometimes added impromptu obstacles—like crawling up a slide or jumping a fence—to keep him amused. When they came home dappled with sweat and sand, Daniela's mother ushered them to the family dinner table, where they joked and chatted over steaming plates of rice, beans, and *pão de queijo* (Brazilian cheese bread).

But everything changed when Daniela lost the first race of the fall season. It was an easy five-kilometer run she'd intended to win. Embarrassed, she approached her coach afterward to discuss strategy for the next meet. He suggested that she do some longer runs on the weekends outside of school. *Time to get serious*, Daniela thought. Determined not to lose a second time, she put a calendar up on her bedroom wall to track her daily mileage. She immediately added five-mile runs on Saturdays and Sundays, and pushed herself even harder at weekday school practices. Her efforts paid off. At the season's second meet, she won by a large margin, earning victory whoops and hugs from her ecstatic teammates. "Keep this up, and you'll have your pick of the litter when it comes to college scholarships," her coach beamed. *College scholarships?* she thought. *I can't stop now.*

As the weather got colder, Daniela started running on the basement treadmill. There, she could monitor her pace on a computerized screen, and Alberto's antics couldn't slow her down. She became increasingly meticulous about her routine. She had to do her weekend runs at exactly 8 a.m. If her mother was doing laundry or Alberto was watching cartoons, she paced around the basement anxiously until they retreated upstairs. *Don't they realize how important this is?* she thought, irritated. Steepening the incline and hastening her pace, she was already breathing hard at the one-mile-mark. But she had to keep going. *Besides,* she thought, *I always feel calmer after a run.*

Slowly, her five-mile weekend runs became six miles, then seven. Each increase felt like the tightening of a vise: *If I do seven miles today, I have to do at least seven tomorrow. Anything less is unacceptable.* To accommodate her escalating weekly mileage, she started canceling plans with friends. She replaced study groups and team dinners with interval training and speed workouts. She fell into bed exhausted each evening. Even Alberto began to worry—why was his sister so tired all the time? And what happened to his obstacle course?

Once tanned and healthy, Daniela lost a little weight and became increasingly pale. She continued eating her mother's fried yucca and plantains but found herself enjoying food less the more she ran. Truth be told, she enjoyed everything less.

Do You Exercise Compulsively?

Daniela is battling compulsive exercise. She is another example of someone who has almost anorexia but not OSFED or un-specified feeding and eating disorder. (Her actual eating hasn't been changed enough for her to be diagnosed.) Are you (or a loved one) struggling with compulsive exercise too? Take the following self-test (table 9), developed by eating disorder researchers Lorin Taranis, Stephen Touyz, and Caroline Meyer, to find out.[5] Although this test cannot tell you whether you have almost anorexia (see chapter 1 for that), it will help you understand whether your attitudes about exercise are prob-

lematic. For immediate feedback, take the test online at www.
jennischaefer.com. To score by hand, check out the instructions
in appendix B.

Compulsive Exercise: Five Key Signs

Researchers at Loughborough University, one of the United
Kingdom's top athletic institutions, designed the Compulsive
Exercise Test to measure the five key signs of compulsive exercise. Many are relevant to Daniela, and some may be relevant
to you.

Rule-Driven Behavior

Do you try to follow strict rules about exercise? Daniela told
herself, for example, *If I run less today than I did yesterday, I am
a failure.* Some people need the structure of a sports team,
Zumba class, or cycling club to get and stay active. But if you
can't take a break every once in a while, or if you find yourself
skipping work, school, or social activities for your mandatory
daily workouts, you might be taking this structure too far. In a
large sample of Australian women, trying to follow specific rules
about exercise was nearly twice as common among those with
eating disorders versus those who were healthy.[6] Breaks are
especially important if you are injured or ill, and they are necessary to promote peak performance. Even 2011 Boston marathon
champ Geoffrey Mutai, who captured the prestigious laurel
wreath by running the fastest marathon ever in just over two
hours, takes every Sunday off to attend church with his family.[7]

Weight-Control Exercise

Is your primary motivation for exercise to burn calories, lose
weight, or reduce the percentage of your body fat? It's fine if

Table 9.
Compulsive Exercise Test

INSTRUCTIONS: Please read each statement and select the number from **0** (never true of you) to **5** (always true of you).	Never true: 0	Rarely true: 1	Sometimes true: 2	Often true: 3	Usually true: 4	Always true: 5
1.	I feel happier and/or more positive after I exercise.						
2.	I exercise to improve my appearance.						
3.	I like my days to be organized and structured, of which exercise is just one part.						
4.	I feel less anxious after I exercise.						
5.	I find exercise a chore.						
6.	If I feel I have eaten too much, I will do more exercise.						
7.	My weekly pattern of exercise is repetitive.						
8.	I do not exercise to be slim.						
9.	If I cannot exercise, I feel low or depressed.						
10.	I feel extremely guilty if I miss an exercise session.						
11.	I usually continue to exercise despite injury, unless I am very ill or too injured.						

12.	I enjoy exercising.					
13.	I exercise to burn calories and lose weight.					
14.	I feel less stressed and/or tense after I exercise.					
15.	If I miss an exercise session, I will try to make up for it when I next exercise.					
16.	If I cannot exercise, I feel agitated and/or irritable.					
17.	Exercise improves my mood.					
18.	If I cannot exercise, I worry that I will gain weight.					
19.	I follow a set routine for my exercise sessions (e.g., walk or run the same route, particular exercises, same amount of time, and so on).					
20.	If I cannot exercise, I feel angry and/or frustrated.					
21.	I do not enjoy exercising.					
22.	I feel like I've let myself down if I miss an exercise session.					
23.	If I cannot exercise, I feel anxious.					
24.	I feel less depressed or low after I exercise.					

Note: The Compulsive Exercise Test has been reproduced with permission. It can be downloaded at www.jennischaefer.com.

appearance is one of many reasons—such as heart health, strength, socializing, or fun. But if you allow yourself to eat only the number of calories that your workout just burned off (an eating disorder behavior called "debting"), or you exercise specifically to torch the calories you just ate (a form of purging), these can be red flags. In her memoir *Diary of an Exercise Addict*, Peach Friedman explained it this way: "When I was an exercise bulimic . . . I felt somehow wrong for eating. I felt fat. I felt full and that made me hate myself. I ran, I swam, I danced, I lifted, I did all of this to get rid of something—of myself."[8] Exercise can be a particularly deceptive method of purging because, unlike vomiting or laxative misuse, it's usually healthy for you. But remember, you still deserve to eat breakfast tomorrow even if you skip your morning spin class.

Mood Improvement

Do you exercise specifically to avoid negative emotions? An old Nike advertisement featured a man jogging above a tagline asking, "Who says you can't run away from your problems?" Although you cannot actually become physiologically addicted to exercise, you may find it psychologically addicting if it's your go-to strategy when you are feeling low. You may feel anxious (like Daniela) or guilty if you are unable to exercise. Or you may even have withdrawal symptoms, such as depression, when you stop or cut back. Your self-worth may become dependent on how much you work out or how hard you push yourself. Although exercise is a natural antidepressant that releases endorphins and increases blood flow to the brain, it's important to have more than one tool in your toolbox when it comes to regulating your emotions.

Lack of Exercise Enjoyment

Do you continue the same exercise routine even if it feels like a chore? For Daniela, running started out as enjoyable and social, but ultimately became monotonous and solitary. If you dread your workouts or beat yourself up for not meeting an unrealistically high standard of athletic achievement, compulsive exercise may be a problem for you. Jenni began exercising during her recovery when her doctor finally said she was healthy enough. In the beginning, going from sedentary to active felt great. But it didn't take long for Ed to apply compulsivity to the mix. When that happened, Jenni no longer looked forward to exercising; instead she saw it as an hour of activity that seemed to dictate the rest of her day. *Change your plans with friends to get your workout in today. Wake up extra early to go to the gym— it doesn't matter if you are tired the rest of the day.*

Exercise Rigidity

Does your exercise routine feel inflexible, rigid, or extreme? Among individuals with eating disorders, those who exercise excessively also exhibit higher levels of perfectionism and obsessive-compulsive personality traits.[9] You may struggle with compulsive exercise if you feel compelled to do the same number of crunches or squats every time you hit the gym or use the same route every time you jog or cycle. Like Daniela, you may need to exercise at the same time each day, feel afraid to vary the types of exercise that you do, or exercise alone to avoid having your routine disturbed. If you are training well beyond the program that your coach or trainer recommends, or you feel you have to "make up for" missed sessions, that is also a red flag. Peach Friedman found that her exercise program became less rigid as her eating disorder receded: "These days, I still work out. . . . But when I'm sick, I rest. And when I don't feel like it, I don't exercise. And when I go on vacation, I chill out and enjoy myself. I'm flexible about the time of day I hit the gym or the road, and I'm flexible, too, about what sort of exercise I'm getting. In fact, the more variety, the better . . . and I'll try anything new."[10]

Medical Complications of Compulsive Exercise

Not only is compulsive exercise related to disordered eating, but it can also be associated with health problems. A study of British Olympians and members of the prestigious 100-marathon club demonstrated that, sometimes, it's possible to do too much of a good thing. Researchers compared lifelong older (ages 50 to 67) and younger (ages 26 to 40) endurance athletes to nonathlete controls of the same age. Half of the older endurance athletes—but none of the younger athletes or control nonathletes—had myocardial fibrosis (a condition in which the heart muscle develops scar tissue that contributes to abnormal heart rhythms).[11] Although this was a cross-sectional study that cannot prove that participation in endurance events caused the heart damage, it nonetheless provides preliminary evidence of a possible dark side to intensive training. To complicate matters, a low resting heart rate, which can be the sign of a healthy athletic heart, can also signal a dangerous eating disorder. If you have a low resting heart rate, you should speak with your doctor about possible causes.

Health problems are even more common when excessive exercise is coupled with disordered eating. In Dr. Thomas's study of adolescent female ballet students, those with a lifetime history of self-induced vomiting were significantly more likely to report dance-related injuries (such as stress fractures, broken bones, and tendinitis) than students who did not report vomiting.[12] And among those with injuries, those who vomited had to take more than twice as many days away from ballet to recuperate. Some of these dancers may have been suffering from the "female athlete triad" of low energy availability (up to and including an eating disorder), menstrual disturbance (up to and including amenorrhea), and bone loss (up to and including osteoporosis).

U.S. Olympic silver medalist in track cycling Dotsie Bausch told us that she wasn't able to become an elite athlete until she fully recovered from her eating disorder. At the age of twenty-one, Dotsie began struggling with anorexia nervosa and compulsive exercise, which she described as "gym insanity," spending "hours and hours on the Stairmaster and elliptical counting every calorie I was burning." Although she finally made peace with food through treatment, her relationship with exercise was more complicated. After two years, "I asked my therapist if I would ever be able to exercise in a healthy way again, because I would not consider myself healed until I could at least move my body in a regular way and enjoy being outside and exercising," she said. To fully heal, her therapist suggested that she try a different type of physical activity—one that wouldn't remind her of her dark days of fasting and purging. Dotsie chose cycling. Rising quickly through the ranks, she made it all the way to the podium at the 2012 Olympic Games in London. "It was the most amazing thing!" she said. "I felt incredibly proud to represent my country."[13]

Not Moving Enough

Compulsive exercise is not the only exercise problem that people with almost anorexia can face: exercise avoidance is also prevalent. In a recent study, only 21 percent of individuals with subclinical eating disorders reported that exercise interfered with other activities, caused distress, continued despite injury, or was excessive.[14] That means 79 percent did not find too much exercise to be a problem. A more insidious, but equally problematic, pattern among individuals with almost anorexia is not exercising enough. And it's easy to see why. If you are very critical of your body, you may skip the gym because you don't want to be seen wearing fitted exercise clothes in public or because you engage in black-and-white thinking around exercise. Have you ever said to yourself, for example, "I totally blew it by eating pizza at lunch today, so there's no point to doing the elliptical tonight"?

Another reason some people avoid exercising is that they buy the idea that they can't settle for anything less than an absolutely grueling workout. For instance, if you believe that each workout session must be a one-hour high-intensity class at the gym, then you might not exercise at all on days when you have only twenty minutes to spare. Instead of not exercising, in those twenty minutes you could simply get outside and enjoy a nice walk around your neighborhood. Dr. Thomas loves to jog along the Charles River with her good friend Luana. Their whole route takes less than thirty minutes, which feels manageable to her even on a hectic workday.

Despite what you read on the covers of popular women's health and exercise magazines, moderate, noncompulsive exercise has many benefits other than helping you "drop a jeans size in 7 days!" Exercise can relieve stress, improve sleep, decrease blood pressure, and reduce heart disease risk. A recent meta-analysis of thirty studies found that exercise is significantly more effective than no intervention and may be just as effective as therapy or antidepressant medication in providing symptom relief for adults with depression.[15] Exercise may even help you

Jenni's Journey

I am more at home on a bicycle than in stilettos. I have had one broken bone in my life and it happened while walking down stairs in high heels—not plummeting to the bottom of a rocky hill on my mountain bike. After breaking my foot, I sported a hard cast and crutches for several months. By the time the doctor removed the cast, my lower leg looked thin, weak, and lifeless. Since Ed was no longer in the picture, I actually couldn't wait to gain the weight back. This is a "180" from my life with Ed when he would have cheered, "Let's try to shrink your other leg now!" (He wouldn't have even minded breaking it to achieve that goal.) But I can now say that being strong feels worlds better than being super-skinny. Learning how to exercise intuitively in recovery helped to shift my focus from what my body looks like to what it can do. I appreciate my body for everything from simply lifting myself out of bed each morning to taking on difficult challenges like ice climbing, which is basically scaling a frozen waterfall with ice picks. When hanging from the ice on the side of a mountain, I guarantee that my concentration is on gratitude for my strong arms and legs—not on what I look like suspended in the harness. My body has incredible healing powers too. Weight-bearing exercise like walking helped to combat the osteoporosis caused by my eating disorder and to bring my bone density back to normal. Now, if only I could get Dr. Thomas to teach me how to walk in heels . . .

reverse some of the negative health consequences of almost anorexia. In one study of women who had struggled with anorexia nervosa, those who engaged in weight-bearing exercise (such as running, soccer, or dance) after achieving full recovery had greater bone mineral density than those who did not exercise at all.[16] In contrast, those who engaged in exercise while still in the throes of their eating disorder had lower bone density compared to those who were sedentary. This suggests that exercise can be beneficial for women recovering from eating disorders—as long as they are medically stable and have achieved a healthy weight. So, even for someone like Daniela, we wouldn't recommend eliminating exercise completely. Instead, we would recommend striking a healthy balance that we like to call "intuitive exercise."

Intuitive Exercise

Put simply, intuitive exercise[17] is the opposite of compulsive exercise. Whereas compulsive exercise is rule-driven, weight-focused, tedious, and rigid, intuitive exercise is rule-free, multifaceted, fun, and flexible. Intuitive exercise means paying attention to and respecting your body sensations and energy levels—sometimes your body wants to ride a bike, and sometimes it craves lying on the couch. Intuitive exercise means picking an exercise activity because you enjoy it, not because it burns the most calories. Clinical psychologist Beth Hartman McGilley has told her patients, "Find a way to move that moves you."[18] If you love yoga, then there's no need to feel guilty about skipping the treadmill. There is even some evidence that yoga may contribute to decreases in disordered eating.[19] Intuitive exercise also means not overdoing it; unless you want to become a professional yoga instructor, there's no need to sign up for the 500-hour teacher training.

The hard part about intuitive exercise is that we live in a world where so many people, including gym teachers, coaches, fitness instructors, and even health care professionals, promote compulsivity when it comes to moving our bodies. Participating in a standard gym class in many ways can be like subjecting yourself to Societal Ed's lies for an hour: "You must work harder to burn off the food you ate last weekend. Get rid of those jiggling thighs for good." It takes knowledge and awareness to combat these messages. We both know from personal experience that healthy thighs are meant to jiggle!

Not all fitness classes are negative. If you decide to join a gym, we recommend that you choose one with a positive environment that focuses on health and fun. A good way to get to know a gym's culture is to work out there a time or two. Most gyms will give prospective members at least one free pass. When you are exercising at a gym, look around. Do the other members trigger you? Are they chiseled, carbon copies of one another? Do fliers on the wall advertise unhealthy weight-loss strategies? When it comes to eating disorders, your environment can make a big difference. For example, Dr. Thomas's research has revealed that adolescent dancers who train at schools affiliated with elite national ballet companies exhibit higher rates of eating disorders than those who train at smaller local or regional centers.[20] So it's worth finding a nontriggering gym!

When you consider your intuitive exercise routine, choose activities that complement your personality. If you like to be social, you might want to join a running or walking group so you can chat while you move. If you have a competitive spirit, enroll in a team sport. People who are more introverted and who want to use their exercise time for solitude and meditation obviously won't want to go walking with a group of chatty women. Instead, they might try gentle hiking or yoga—both activities that can be done in groups but also give you time to reflect inward. Get creative with your exercise. Some places offer dance classes where you can learn the choreography to a Broadway musical. You may find a belly dancing class or invest in a hula hoop or jump rope.

Daniela's Intuitive Exercise Program

After Daniela developed a stress fracture in her ankle, her mother began to worry and spoke with her coach. Her coach had also noticed both that Daniela's performance was declining and that she had trained through the pain for several weeks, so he decided to talk to her about compulsive overtraining. He encouraged Daniela to look honestly at what she was doing to her body and to make some positive changes. At first, Daniela was reluctant to reduce her weekly mileage. She worried that if she took rest days, she would lose her edge, and that—although she was at a normal weight—her muscle would "melt into fat." When her coach suggested that Daniela consider cross-training with different types of exercise, Daniela felt defensive: "Running is my coping skill," she explained. After taking the Compulsive Exercise Test and identifying the elements of her training program that were potentially problematic, Daniela set the following goals:

1. Run a maximum of three to four times per week

2. Limit mileage to that recommended by her coach (typically less than four miles at a time)

3. No canceling social activities (like dinner with friends) to exercise

4. Cross-train with other low-impact activities (such as yoga or Zumba on off days)

5. Take two rest days (no exercise at all) per week

6. Practice improving mood with non-exercise activities (for example, phone a friend, watch a funny video, play with Alberto)

Lifestyle Activity

Practicing intuitive exercise also means balancing formal exercise with any informal exercise you do throughout the day. Lifestyle activity includes any unstructured movement that you do in the course of daily life, such as walking to work, tidying your home, raking the yard, or running after toddlers.

Lifestyle activity is important in the context of almost anorexia for two reasons. First, depending on the intensity, it can partly or even entirely take the place of formal exercise. If you are a military service member who must stay deployment-ready, a mail carrier who walks miles per day making deliveries, or a sales clerk who is constantly moving around to help customers, there may be little need to incorporate structured exercise into your day. Similarly, Daniela didn't need to add extra workouts to her already intense cross-country practices. Second, individuals with almost anorexia and other eating disorders are vulnerable to engaging in excessive lifestyle activity. One of Dr. Thomas's patients put his computer on top of a cardboard box so that he could stand at his desk all day at work, and another couldn't stop fidgeting to burn calories during appointments. At the height of Jenni's illness, Ed loved that she took jobs as a waitress, auditorium usher, and security guard so that she had to walk and stand all day. Animal studies provide clues to the counterintuitive link between malnutrition and physical activity. In a model called "activity-based anorexia," mice and rats who are given very limited access to food and unlimited access to a running wheel will literally run themselves to death.[21] Researchers speculate that this excessive wheel running may have evolutionary roots in migratory behavior, which would have been adaptive for starving animals who needed to move on to a new habitat with more plentiful food. But luckily none of us are experimental lab mice, so it's important to consider lifestyle activity when selecting our structured exercise activities.

Your Intuitive Exercise Schedule

Whether you are exercising too much or too little, making an exercise plan for the week can be a great first step to finding balance. In table 10, Jenni has shared a sample exercise schedule for a typical week while she was working on this book. Notice how she incorporates several features of intuitive exercise into her routine. First, her schedule is flexible; it includes a variety of activities (from volleyball to mountain biking), rather than just one. Second, she takes rest days. She's a writer, so her lifestyle involves plenty of sitting down, and that's okay. Third, she incorporates social exercise, like going for a "wog" (combined walk/run) with Dr. Thomas. Fourth, she counts lifestyle activity as exercise. Her mountain biking date might not have been the most strenuous cycling experience (after all, she was

Table 10.

Jenni's Intuitive Exercise Schedule

Monday	Tuesday	Wednesday	Thursday	Friday	Saturday	Sunday
11 a.m. Yoga class at new studio that just opened up by my house (60 minutes)	Rest (writing outside on my picnic table)	6:30 p.m. Intramural volleyball game with my fellow Texas A&M alums in Austin —Go Aggies! (30 minutes)	5 p.m. Bike ride on hilly trail—first date with new guy. It's a good sign that we both like mountain biking! (50 minutes)	Walking through the Austin and Boston airports carrying heavy bags. Excited to visit Dr. Thomas to work on book. (20 minutes)	Rest (writing book on Dr. Thomas's couch)	3 p.m. "Wogging" with Dr. Thomas around Charles River esplanade to boost creativity (30 minutes)

This week's total (minutes): ___190___

hanging out with a new guy!), but it still counts as activity. Likewise, walking around an airport with heavy luggage is included on her schedule. Lastly, she meets the surgeon general's recommendation of at least 150 minutes of physical activity weekly, but she doesn't push herself too far. To make your own intuitive exercise plan, use table 11 or write your plan in a notebook.

Depending on your current relationship with exercise, you might be able to jump right into creating your own intuitive program. But first be sure to consult with a health care professional and to take a look at some basic guidelines below:

- Make a list of indoor exercise activities that you enjoy. You don't need to join a gym for intuitive exercise. Many exercise classes are available for free online or even on mobile apps. And don't forget that you are born with everything you need to exercise: your body.

- Make a list of outdoor activities that get your body moving—and that you like. These might include walking, jogging, riding a bicycle, swimming in a local pool, or bumping a volleyball with a friend.

- Think about friends or family members who might want to join in on some of these activities. Talk with them about their availability. Compare schedules.

Now, let's get to your intuitive exercise schedule (table 11):

- Begin by scheduling rest days to make sure you get them in. We recommend including at least two per week.

Table 11.
Your Intuitive Exercise Schedule

Monday	Tuesday	Wednesday	Thursday	Friday	Saturday	Sunday

This week's total (minutes): _____

continued on next page

Table 11 continued

Intuitive exercise means . . .

- Your exercise routine is flexible. You do a variety of activities that are driven by how your body feels, not by rules.

- The "why" behind exercise is not entirely about controlling your weight. You exercise for a variety of reasons, including having fun, socializing, and maintaining good health.

- Missing an exercise opportunity does not influence your mood in a negative way.

- Exercise is not a chore. When you are active, you select activities that you enjoy.

- You want to. There is no "have to" in regard to when and how much you exercise.

- You account for unstructured or "lifestyle" physical activity when planning structured exercise.

- You eat enough food to adequately fuel your level of physical activity.

This exercise can be downloaded at www.almostanorexic.com.

- Add exercise activities that you will do with a friend or family member.
- Add exercises that you will do by yourself.
- Be flexible. Adjust your schedule as needed based on how your body feels.
- Enjoy. Don't forget that exercise is supposed to be fun.

9

Accepting and Loving Your Body
(Yes, We Said Loving!)

Even though you cannot escape Societal Ed's emphasis on appearance, with a little effort, you can absolutely change your own focus. You might not believe us now—and that's okay—but it is possible to shift your perspective. Learning to love your body means forgoing fat talk, ceasing body checking, and escaping from body hiding. Full freedom does not mean that you will never have a negative thought about your body. It does mean that you can get to a place where you no longer base your entire self-worth on the number on the scale. From time to time, you might hear Societal Ed, who tells all of us to eat less and lose weight. But thanks to your hard work, you will be in a far better position to cope with Societal Ed's pressures than those who have never struggled with disordered eating. You can learn to be healthier and happier than you might have otherwise been.

Replace Fat Talk with Phat Talk

Fat talk is ubiquitous. Sometimes we participate without even realizing it. As clinical psychologist Cynthia Bulik highlighted in *Woman in the Mirror*, there are many different kinds of fat talk—ranging from *can't-take-a-compliment fat talk* ("Someone says, 'You look absolutely stunning tonight.' You say, 'Thank God for Spanx!'") to *stealth fat talk* ("You must be spending lots of time at the gym." Translation: "You looked really out of shape before)."[1] Unfortunately, all types of fat talk can be harmful. In one experiment, just hearing a peer engage in fat talk (saying, "Ugh, look at her thighs" in response to a magazine advertisement) increased listeners' own guilt and body dissatisfaction.[2]

The best thing you can do with fat talk is quit. Cold turkey. Delta Delta Delta sorority created Fat Talk Free® Week. During the week, they have encouraged college students to sign the following pledge:

> "Today I promise to End Fat Talk™ in conversations with my friends, my family, and myself. Starting now, I will strive not for a thin-ideal but for a healthy ideal, which I know looks different for every person, and focuses on health not weight or size. I will celebrate the things about myself and the people in my life that have nothing to do with how we look."[3]

But you don't have to be a college student to take the pledge. Every week is free of fat talk at Dr. Thomas's house. Jenni's too. Sign your name now, here in the book, or make a pledge on a separate piece of paper and display it somewhere where you will see it daily.

Today I will not engage in "fat talk."

Signed, _____

For a while, you might need to recommit to this pledge each day. Once you've changed the conversation for yourself, see how you can have an impact on those around you. Dr. Thomas does not allow fat talk in her therapy groups. Jenni once saw a sign hanging up in an office that said, "Thank you for not talking about your diet. Please be considerate of others . . . please do not obsess about your weight in this area." Brilliant. Others have asked friends and colleagues to put money in a mason jar every time they accidentally participate in fat talk. After a while, you may have enough money to buy something special for yourself or to donate to a good cause.

We realize that changing the conversation is difficult. Dr. Thomas tries hard not to reinforce appearance concerns by complimenting her patients' choice of outfits, even though she loves fashion. This is where "phat talk" comes in. *Phat* (pronounced "fat") is a slang term from the 1990s, which loosely translates to "cool." When you connect with others, rather than focusing on appearance as an opening line ("You look great!"), comment on another positive quality. For example, you can say, "You seem really happy" or "I'm so glad to see you." With young children, in particular, you might have noticed that people tend to comment on outward appearance first by saying something like, "You are so cute." What might happen if a generation of little girls grew up hearing "You are so smart" instead? In a wildly popular *Huffington Post* blog entry entitled "How to Talk to Little Girls," journalist Lisa Bloom suggested, "Try this the next time you meet a little girl.

She may be surprised and unsure at first, because few ask her about her mind, but be patient and stick with it. Ask her what she's reading. What does she like and dislike, and why? There are no wrong answers. You're just generating an intelligent conversation that respects her brain. For older girls, ask her about current events issues: pollution, wars, school budgets slashed. What bothers her out there in the world? How would she fix it if she had a magic wand? You may get some intriguing answers. Tell her about your ideas and accomplishments and your favorite books. Model for her what a thinking woman says and does."[4]

These strategies may be helpful for reducing the fat talk that is happening out loud around you. But what about the fat talk going on inside your own head? That was an area where Meredith suffered immensely.

Meredith

FAT, Meredith read the word yet again, carved into the inside of her left arm as she waited for her friend Matt to pick her up for a movie. Even though she wholeheartedly believed the word described her, she really wished that she hadn't done that or at least had chosen a more inconspicuous spot. She felt so ashamed when people saw it, which happened a lot, especially when playing guitar at her favorite coffee shop. Recalling how the pain of the sharp edge against her skin felt so much better than her deep, dark inside, she distinctly remembered why she had done it: she hated her body. Still, she vowed never to cut again, and she hasn't. But Meredith's destructive behaviors didn't stop—or even start—there.

Her "drug" of choice was really food and had been for as

long as she could remember. The earliest memory she can recall is at six years old, a time when she was sexually abused at the hand of a person her parents called a "close friend." *Why did he choose me?* Meredith wondered. With the mind of a child, she could only decipher that her early-developing breasts and curvy body must have been the reason. Maybe that's why she was the only girl in her school getting abused. Or at least that's what she thought. So, naturally, she did anything she could think of to look smaller and younger—less like a woman. *I won't eat. Then maybe he will stop.* A welcome side effect of restricting her eating was not feeling much either. The pain of the abuse was so horrendous that Meredith's young mind couldn't even acknowledge it. All that she could really get in touch with was the echoing message *It's your fault*, and she despised herself for it.

Long after her abuser had moved away and even after Meredith had left home and began studying music at a great college, this message of blame festered in her head. She was willing to try anything to make the pain go away. What seemed to work best was restricting food and cutting back on liquids as well. When she restricted, her world seemed much simpler. It was as if her brain could only hold a certain amount of information on the limited fuel, and when she was lucky, it didn't obsess about the past.

Since restricting food couldn't erase her self-described "disgusting" feminine shape, she took additional measures, including wearing sports bras (that bound her breasts tightly), loose jeans, and sweatshirts. *Men won't want me now*, she thought. Matt was someone who was interested in dating her, but he had long since given up on that chance, especially after she had alarmed him by being so startled by his invitation to prom years earlier. Now he just appreciated her friendship.

When he pulled alongside the curb in front of her apartment building, he winced at her ever-shrinking body. Meredith was only slightly underweight, but Matt had seen the progression, including her pale skin and dull eyes, and he was worried—still. They had discussed her eating behaviors before, and now she had even reached a point where she wanted to change. It was the purging. Although she made herself throw up only about once a week after eating very small meals, she hated the feeling of being out of control. She would do anything to stop purging. Still, she was vehemently opposed to seeking professional help. Matt couldn't help but look at *FAT* on her arm when she shut the car door and her sleeve rode up. Meredith noticed that he was looking, so in the already awkward moment, Matt said, "I'm concerned, Mer. What if I help you find a therapist? Would you go just once?"

Wrapped in an extra sweatshirt to stay warm, Meredith stewed it over during the entire three-hour movie, as she watched people enjoying popcorn and candy seemingly guilt-free. Finally, upon leaving, she looked at Matt and said, "Okay." He knew what she meant and sent her a text the next day: "www.jenniferjthomasphd.com. Proud of you."

Walking into Dr. Thomas's office a few days later felt surreal to Meredith. Before long she was diagnosed with purging disorder—and wondering how the stars had aligned so that she actually ended up in therapy. Just as she sat down in the comfy couch across from Dr. Thomas, a voice in Meredith's head said, *Talk about anything—except that.* As the weeks went by, Meredith did finally open up about her history of being abused.

But when she spoke about what happened, Meredith appeared to be a news reporter telling a story—no emotion.

In one session, knowing Meredith's passion for music, Dr. Thomas played a song, "She Blames Herself" from Jenni's CD *phoenix, Tennessee*. Meredith listened, and for the first time in therapy, shed a tear, releasing just a little of the shame.

> *She blames herself she blames it all*
> *On how she dressed the way she walked*
> *Drowning in shame and so much guilt*
> *Who can she trust who can she tell*
> *When she's too scared to even ask for help*
> *It was all his fault and still*
> *She blames herself* [5]

Meredith resonated with the song and felt just a little lighter—not in pounds but in self-hate. This emotion was a starting place for Dr. Thomas to help Meredith direct her anger appropriately—outward, not inward. Along with working through the abuse, they focused on normalizing her eating. This included bringing water and snacks to eat in some sessions where she felt safe. At first, Meredith wanted Dr. Thomas to simply help her stop purging. But Meredith eventually realized that getting better meant improving in all areas regarding food. She finally stopped both purging and restricting but still didn't feel safe in her body. Only after she worked through her trauma did she feel she deserved to improve her body image. In the beginning, they worked on decreasing her body checking and avoidance behaviors. Meredith even brought Dr. Thomas her entire collection of tape measures and belts that she had been secretly using to monitor her body size. Although she handed over the collection, at first she was not willing to completely give up these items, so Dr. Thomas kept them in a drawer in her office. As the months went by, Meredith forgot about the drawer. When she finally remembered, she couldn't believe that she had forgotten. At this point, she gave Dr. Thomas full permission to get rid of them—each and every one.

Slowly, Meredith was able to make similar progress with wearing more normal clothes. As with her changes in eating, Meredith began by taking small steps. At first, she just experimented with wearing shorts and even skirts to therapy sessions. In time, she was able to incorporate this attire into her everyday life. Ultimately, Dr. Thomas and Meredith moved toward mirror exposure therapy. Standing in front of a full-length mirror, Meredith practiced describing herself in neutral, objective terms, instead of using Ed's self-deprecating language. No longer constrained by the loaded terms of *fat* and *ugly*, she started noticing positive features of her body, like her big green eyes, delicate fingers, and muscular calves. Today, when Meredith plays guitar, she doesn't mind showing that scar on her arm—it's fading more and more each day. She smiles, genuinely happy in her life—and her body. And Matt, her *boyfriend*, attends all of her shows.

Some theorize that victims of sexual abuse either gain or lose weight as a form of protection or that they harm their bodies because of intense shame. Meredith hoped that her thin body, lacking hips and breasts, would divert unwanted male attention, and she cut herself as a form of self-punishment. Although research in this area is limited and has not proven that people unconsciously or consciously lose and/or gain weight or harm themselves for this reason, if you have experienced a trauma, you might connect with this idea. (We recommend that you talk to a professional about the trauma if you have not done so already.) Indeed, research suggests there is a modest association between childhood sexual abuse and both eating disorders and self-harm behaviors such as cutting.[6] Regardless of the reason you struggle with poor body image, there are several techniques that are likely to help reduce your distress.

Stop Body Checking

Meredith truly wrestled with body checking. You may recall that Dante (who compulsively measured his bicep muscles) and Abriana (who pinched her thighs in front of the mirror) struggled with this as well. Research suggests a strong connection between body checking and poor body image. In one study, women without eating disorders were instructed to scrutinize their most disliked body parts in the mirror for fifteen minutes. Compared to a control group, the women who body checked reported feeling fatter, more self-critical, and more dissatisfied with their bodies.[7] The main reason body checking is so detrimental is that it gives you distorted information about what you really look like.

When it comes to body checking, are you giving extra attention to some inconsequential body feature, like a teeny dimple on your stomach, when the overall picture that others see is a strong and healthy body? Selective attention can skew your perception and cause you to miss things. In a classic study of a phenomenon called "inattentional blindness," participants were asked to count the passes between basketball players wearing black shirts versus those wearing white shirts.

They were so intent on counting the passes against the complex choreography of dribbling and dodging that half of them didn't even notice a person wearing a gorilla costume walking across the scene. This was true even when the gorilla stopped in the middle of the scene, faced the camera, and thumped its chest![8] It's amazing how much we miss when we are not expecting to see it.

Even worse, when you repeat the same body checking behaviors every day (or hour, or minute!), you already know which "flaws" to look for. As a young person, you may have read *Where's Waldo*, a children's book series that asks kids to scan complex scenes to find a man named Waldo, who is wearing a distinctive beanie hat and striped shirt. These books are fun at first—until you figure out where Waldo is on each page. Then they get a little boring. Body checking is like that. Once you've found your "flaws," you are no longer gaining new information; you are just reinforcing—not to mention magnifying—your already negative self-view.

Another reason you may be getting poor information from shape checking is that people are not very good at detecting visual change. Demonstrating a phenomenon that psychologists call "change blindness," college students were asked to view and summarize a brief movie clip of a man answering a telephone. In the clip, the sole actor was replaced with a similar-looking and similarly dressed actor in between scenes. Of the forty participants, only 33 percent noticed the change in actors![9] Similarly, Dr. Thomas usually hopes that her husband will compliment her when she gets a manicure. Even though he's a great guy, he doesn't always notice. It's the same with our bodies. The shape changes for which you might be checking are likely to be very subtle—barely detectable by yourself, let alone anyone else. Furthermore, there is an element of physiological impossibility in body checking. Given that you'd need to consume many hundreds of calories more than you burn in order to gain even one pound, it's not even possible to do this in just a few minutes' time.

The bottom line? We strongly encourage you to step away from the skinny jeans. Refraining from scrutinizing himself in the gym mirror was what helped Dante to get better. (Yes, he eventually sought help.) We know changing this behavior isn't easy, so we've provided a list of strategies below. You can remember these strategies with the acronym OLD. "O" is for *obstruction* strategies that will make checking less automatic. For example, if you throw away your scale, it will be harder for you to weigh yourself. "L" is for techniques that *limit* the amount of time you spend in high-risk situations for checking, like standing in front of the bathroom mirror. Lastly, "D" is for *delay* and *distract*. This means engaging in alternative activities while you wait for the body checking urge to diminish. To see how Meredith ultimately overcame tape measure and mirror checking, check out table 12. Then, take the time to fill out table 13 for yourself, or use a notebook to record the personal strategies you will try.

Table 12.
Meredith's Body Checking Is Getting OLD

Checking behavior to be reduced: (such as pinching for fatness, weighing, trying on too-small clothes) *Using tape measure and mirror to determine size of my waist and legs*		
Behavioral strategies for reducing body checking:		
Obstruct (for example, get rid of tape measure, throw away too-small jeans)	**Limit** (for example, limit mirror use to socially normal times, such as getting dressed in morning or brushing teeth at night)	**Delay and Distract** (for example, set timer for 15 minutes to see if urge decreases; keep hands busy with stress ball)
Give tape measure to Dr. Thomas; move full-length mirror from bedroom into closet	*Stop staring at myself in the full-length mirror before bed, analyzing the size of my waist and legs. Only use mirror for 5 minutes while washing face and brushing teeth.*	*If I feel the urge to go to the store and buy a tape measure or to use something else to measure myself, set a timer for 15 minutes. Call Matt or another friend while waiting for the timer to ring.*

Table 13.
Your Body Checking Is Getting OLD

Checking behavior to be reduced:
(such as pinching for fatness, weighing, trying on too-small clothes)

Behavioral strategies for reducing body checking:		
Obstruct (for example, get rid of tape measure, throw away too-small jeans)	**Limit** (for example, limit mirror use to socially normal times, such as getting dressed in morning or brushing teeth at night)	**Delay and Distract** (for example, set timer for 15 minutes to see if urge decreases; keep hands busy with stress ball)

This exercise can be downloaded at www.almostanorexic.com.

Change the Conversation with Your Mirror

Do you scrutinize yourself in the mirror? As Meredith and Dante know all too well, mirror scrutiny is a special type of body checking. One of the most effective ways to overcome this is to practice using the mirror differently. A treatment called "mirror exposure therapy" can help.

In mirror exposure, you stand in front of a full-length mirror but, rather than scrutinizing individual body parts and engaging in harsh self-criticism (as in body checking), you practice scanning your entire body and making neutral and descriptive statements. For example, instead of staring first at your stomach, then at your thighs, and calling yourself names like "fat," "disgusting," or "gross," you would focus on every part of your body in turn, describing your hair color, eye color, skin texture, and more. To come up with neutral statements, you can ask yourself, *How might I describe my appearance so that a stranger could easily pick me out of a crowd?* If you use words like *fat* or *ugly*, the stranger would be completely unable to distinguish you from other individuals with almost anorexia, who sadly would describe themselves exactly the same way. In contrast, if you use neutral descriptors (such as brown hair, blue eyes, light brown skin), the stranger would have a much easier time identifying you. Try it at home on your own. If you are skeptical or reluctant, know that you are not alone. Dr. Sherrie Delinsky told us, "The biggest stumbling blocks to mirror exposure are anxiety, which tends to dissipate quickly and with practice, and lack of language. For the latter problem, I suggest that individuals ask others for suggestions or brainstorm non-judgmental terms that can be used to describe one's physical appearance, especially focusing on texture, color, symmetry, shape, and proportion. I have had patients who practice this technique tell me, 'I don't look nearly as bad as I thought,' 'I am much more proportionate than I thought,' and 'Wow, I need to be much nicer to myself.'"[10] In one study, which Dr. Delinsky coauthored, women with almost anorexia and other officially recognized eating disorders showed greater decreases in body checking, body dissatisfaction, and eating disorder symptoms after completing five sessions of mirror exposure therapy compared to a control group who did not receive this treatment.[11]

If changing your self-talk language from critical to neutral does not come easily to you, consider connecting with someone who can help you develop a list of descriptors. Write the terms you choose on a note and attach it to your bathroom mirror to remind yourself about the power of mirror exposure therapy. Over time, take this to a new level: begin posting compliments for yourself and others on the reflective surfaces in your home, school, grocery store, or gym, as motivational speaker Caitlyn Boyle describes in her book and blog *Operation Beautiful*.[12] Dr. Thomas loves looking in the mirrors at the residential treatment program where she conducts her research. There are always positive messages on posters, sticky notes, and collages: *You are beautiful! Your smile is gorgeous! There's something all over your face—oh wait, it must be a whole bunch of beautiful! Justin Bieber loves girls who eat breakfast!* Try putting a positive note in your own bathroom. (If you don't have "Bieber Fever," you can insert your own celebrity crush.)

We appreciate that this may feel like a mixed message *(Don't worry about how you look, but tell yourself how beautiful you are)*. You might want to look your best, and that's okay— it's natural. What's important is that you don't sacrifice your quality of life and your happiness to achieve a specific look. Remember your self-evaluation pie chart from chapter 5? You want a variety of domains contributing to your self-esteem. All of your time and energy cannot be channeled into shape and weight. Or, rather, it can be. But that wouldn't be a good plan for a happy life.

Stop Comparing (and Despairing!)

Do you frequently compare yourself to others? You are not alone. When looking at Facebook photos, 44 percent of users in one study wished they had the same body or weight as a friend, 32 percent said they feel sad when comparing photos of themselves to their friends', and 37 percent feel that they actually need to change specific parts of their body as a result of this comparing.[13] Not only are we matching ourselves up to other people; we are also comparing ourselves to the bodies we had at different times in our lives. *Can I still fit into my high school cheerleading uniform? Football jersey?* Continual advances in photo-sharing technology make this kind of obsessing ever easier. In fact, in that study, 53 percent of Facebook users said they had compared their body and weight in photos taken at different times during their lives.

Research tells us that comparing leads to despairing. In one study, women (both with and without eating disorder symptoms) experienced greater body dissatisfaction, guilt, and thoughts of dieting after comparing themselves to someone they thought was more attractive than themselves.[14] But we don't really need the research numbers to know that. We have all felt it at one time or another. For example, as a kid growing up in Southern California, Dr. Thomas felt self-conscious about her looks. She had fair skin and dark hair, and so didn't really fit the "California girl" mold in a sea of tanned blonds. Soon Dr. Thomas's new East Coast college classmates were telling her "but you don't look like you're from California." Ultimately, she realized that her unique, high-contrast look has its advantages—it's the perfect frame for red lipstick!

So, if possible, stop comparing. Of course, this might take some time. On your way to achieving a comparison-free zone, begin by trying to at least reduce the bias in your comparisons. Whom do you match yourself up with? Is it usually thin people or others with eating disorders? You might notice that you most often line yourself up against a very specific type of person, especially those who are thinner, younger, and unusually attractive. In recovery, Jenni learned to not compare her insides with another person's outsides. She also learned to stop comparing outsides to outsides and insides to insides, and she still does her best to not compare altogether.

Jenni's Journey

I was an Olympic ice skater as a kid. On the driveway, I imagined that my roller skates became figure-skate blades and the concrete became a sheet of ice. Sometimes, just before completing the difficult triple-lutz jump, I would catch a glance of my short, fat shadow on the driveway. Instantly, the ice melted. But on other days when that gray silhouette appeared tall and skinny, I won the gold. Making comparisons was my mood regulator, an "I'm okay" meter. Unfortunately, the meter tended to sway in the "I'm not okay" direction. When I looked at my older brother's

CONTINUED ON NEXT PAGE

CONTINUED FROM PREVIOUS PAGE

legs next to mine as a kid, comparing led me to wonder, *Why is he skinnier than me? I should be smaller. I'm the little sister.* (I was smaller.) Comparing—and despairing—played a large role in my struggle with disordered eating. In group therapy with other women, the meter was always in full swing, leading me to ask, *Am I the thinnest?* which equated to *Am I the sickest?* and then to *Do I even deserve to be here?* At one point during my recovery, my body became "puffy." My therapist said that lots of people go through this puffy stage when they begin to make true progress with eating, but the other women in my group never looked puffy to me (or at least the meter never registered that). It's not fair, I thought. I felt awful. But, gratefully, the pain of "puffy" pushed me into a place of health where my brain was finally nourished and I could think more clearly. Little by little, I was able to remove my Ed glasses, which, as it turns out, had been magnifying those destructive comparisons all along. I did my best to stop comparing so much—both to others and to previous versions of myself. (I didn't always have cellulite, but I don't mind it today!) At my ideal "Jenni weight," I am my own unique size—one where I have enough energy to laugh, be creative, and even to ice skate again. And just like when I was a kid, I still don't need any actual ice: I complete the triple lutz every time—in Rollerblades these days.

Reducing Avoidance

"Don't wear fitted pants. Don't go out on a date," Ed demands. And to some he says, "Don't even bother leaving your house." Why? His answer is usually something along the lines of "because you are fat" or possibly "unlovable." Obeying Ed just reinforces the negative message that your body should be hidden. Give yourself a chance to prove Ed wrong. Make some changes and, in the process, take your life back.

Ditch Your Sweatpants; Grab Your Swimsuit

If you truly can't imagine not avoiding, try this: avoid avoidance. We know it's not that simple, but change does start with a decision to move in a different direction. Think about an item of clothing in your closet that you use specifically to hide your body. Maybe it's a large sweatshirt or a pair of baggy jeans. Make a commitment to give that item to a trusted friend or a helping professional. As in Meredith's story, ask this person to hang on to it until you are ready to let go completely. What might seem even more challenging is to find a replacement item. For Jenni, the most difficult item of clothing to purchase and to actually wear was a pair of shorts. During early recovery, she had decided that she would never own a pair of shorts again. That seemed easier than facing her fear of wearing them. But today, living in the sweltering summer heat of Austin, Texas, she is quite grateful that she finally bought a pair. Not wearing shorts would have been more difficult in the long run. Now Jenni has shorts of all kinds. Her favorite, of course, are made for biking. It's not about shorts—it's about living. If you decide to challenge yourself to wear a certain item of clothing, you can start with only one hour (or even less) and add on time from there. Remember the dietary experiment in the last chapter? Try that out with body avoidance too. Are you avoiding people, places, or activities in addition to clothes? Try designing an experiment that puts you one step closer to living the life you want to live. As motivational speaker Jessica Weiner entitled her popular body image book, *Life Doesn't Begin 5 Pounds from Now.*[15]

Retail Therapy for Your Almost Anorexic Wardrobe

Anyone who knows Dr. Thomas knows that she loves to shop. (She and her mother-in-law haven't missed a Black Friday sale in almost ten years. True fact.) But that's not why she recommends "retail therapy" to so many of her patients. The real reason she urges them to shop is that, if you struggle with almost anorexia, you probably have an almost anorexic wardrobe to match. The weight fluctuations that accompany disordered eating give a whole new meaning to the phrase "I don't have a thing to wear." Just opening your closet door can unleash a Pandora's box of criticism. "Maybe you should fast today so you can wear me by next week," your skinny jeans quip. "I guess you're stuck with me again today," your long shapeless dress sighs. Between "someday clothes" (those that fit you when you were thinner) and "fat clothes" (those you make yourself wear on bad body image days), you may have very few items in your closet that fit your body—just as it is right now. Typically, the biggest roadblocks to cultivating a non-eating-disorder wardrobe are letting go of ill-fitting clothing that has sentimental value and facing the emotions that accompany buying new clothes that fit you at your current size.

The main reason that letting go of too-small clothing is so difficult is not just that you will miss that particular item or that you spent a lot of money on it. At a deeper level, the pain usually stems from letting go of the perfect person you thought you'd become once you were thin. Blogger Kate Harding calls this "The Fantasy of Being Thin." According to Harding, "The Fantasy of Being Thin is not just about becoming small enough to be perceived as more acceptable. It is about becoming an *entirely different person*—one with far more courage, confidence, and luck than the 'fat you' has. It's not just, 'When I'm thin, I'll look good in a bathing suit'; it's 'When I'm thin, I will be the kind of person who struts down the beach in a bikini, making men weep.'"[16] Remember, like Jenni always says, and sings, "It's Okay to Be Happy":

> *When I lose ten pounds*
> *And then lose five more*
> *When I'm finally size six*
> *Better yet size four*
> *When I grow my hair*
> *To where it should be*
> *When I look in the mirror*
> *And like what I see*
> *Maybe then maybe then maybe then I'll be happy.*[17]

By the end of the song, the message is very clear that you can actually be happy right now. No need to wait for it. When you let go of the fantasy of being thin, you'll travel a long way in reinforcing the belief that it's okay to be happy for yourself. Many of Dr. Thomas's patients have worked toward this goal by turning their too-small jeans or T-shirts into purses, recovery scrapbooks, and more.

Then comes the fun part—buying clothes that truly fit! Angela Liddon, who has written about her eating disorder recovery, started the "Size Healthy" movement to encourage her readers to stop obsessing about the size written on their clothing tags. According to Angela, "Since I recovered from disordered eating, I have tried to stay away from numbers. I never liked the number on clothing. It is so inconsistent and it varies so much by the store. I could walk into a clothing store and leave upset because I wasn't the size I thought I should be." One day, she had a brainstorm: "I know that the size my body is at today, is the size it should be. . . . I thought it would be a really fun idea to write this message [Size Healthy] on my pants! I took a black permanent marker and went to town. It was actually really liberating and fun."[18] Lots of Dr. Thomas's patients have reclaimed their clothing by crossing out the number on the tag and writing "size healthy" instead. You can too.

Jenni described a similar idea in *Goodbye Ed, Hello Me*. During the weight restoration of her treatment, she asked her mom to take her shopping and then cut out the size tags. *Voilà*—a sizeless closet! When using retail therapy to build a non-eating-disorder wardrobe, remember to pick a friendly and age-appropriate store (that is, not a kids or maternity shop, unless you are a child or pregnant). Try bringing multiple sizes in the fitting room so that one ill-fitting item does not feel like a catastrophe. When trying on the clothes, challenge yourself to determine which item really works best for your body before looking at the size tag. And remember to try on entire outfits. Trying on a pair of pants without a top to match will only encourage you to nitpick your supposed "problem areas" instead of seeing your whole self, as others will.

Last to Leave?

You may recall that Jenni's story at the beginning of this book described her negative body image at age four. Not surprisingly, negative body image was the last part of her eating disorder to leave. Even though it took a while, it did go. For some with almost anorexia, the body changes far more quickly than the mind. This means that for a while you might find yourself in a place where your body is healthy but you feel really bad about it. Don't get discouraged. Time and patience go a long way. Longitudinal follow-up studies of individuals with eating disorders suggest that body image is one of the last symptoms to resolve in the recovery process, but that it can and does improve with time.[19] Getting to this healthy place will require support from others.

10

It's Not Just You and Ed
Creating a Circle of Support

Life with almost anorexia is lonely. When your primary relationship is with Ed, there isn't much room left for anyone else. The paradox is that healing inevitably requires reaching out to friends, family, and often professionals. Cultivating this circle of support may require facing your greatest fears, but it is a critical step toward healing.

The Catch-22 of Social Support

When Jenni was sick, she did not feel deeply connected with anyone outside of her immediate family. She talked with some friends on a casual basis, but these relationships lacked depth. Research suggests that people with almost anorexia and other officially recognized eating disorders spend more time performing solitary activities (like doing homework or watching television) and less time socializing with friends than those without eating disorders.[1] Perhaps not surprisingly, then, disordered eating is associated with loneliness.[2] For people who have difficulty eating, socializing can be difficult in a society where we celebrate nearly every holiday and special occasion with food. On an even deeper level, individuals who struggle with disordered eating often have difficulty connecting with other people because of their negative beliefs, such as an intense fear that others will evaluate them negatively, and an extremely fragile sense of self.[3] These concerns may lead to self-protective behaviors—such as not approaching new people, not accepting social invitations, and spending more time alone—that only intensify their feelings of aloneness.

The catch-22 is that greater social support (that is, the emotional and physical comfort we receive from being part of a network of family, friends, and others who care about us) is robustly associated with better mental and physical health. Being close with friends and family might even protect you against the ravages of Ed while you continue to struggle with disordered eating. In a longitudinal study of Australian women with symptoms of a subclinical eating disorder, greater social support predicted better quality of life three years later, even when eating disorder symptoms persisted.[4]

I Want Support, But . . .

If you have not yet told anyone about your struggles with food, Ed probably has a list of reasons why you shouldn't. But as you know by now, Ed has a track record of being wrong. Let's take a closer look at the accuracy of his reasoning.

Everyone Will Judge You

Individuals with almost anorexia and other officially recognized eating disorders typically cite stigma and shame as key barriers to seeking help.[5] Ed may have told you that everyone will judge your drive for thinness as "shallow," your purging behaviors as "disgusting," or your food rules as "crazy," but don't believe it. When Jenni finally confided in her loved ones, no one responded negatively. In fact, many said they admired her more for being honest about her eating disorder than for her "on paper" achievements, like being high school salutatorian or getting accepted to medical school. And consider this: if someone is insensitive enough to judge you for seeking a solution to your eating problem, do you really want to give that person a place in your life?

You Will Just Burden Others

Alternatively, you may be afraid to ask for help because you don't want to "be a bother." Commonly, people who struggle with disordered eating believe that they should be able to recover on their own.[6] If this describes you, try reversing the situation: How would you feel if someone close to you asked you for help with something important? You would probably feel honored and happy to assist. Being trusted and needed feels good. Furthermore, your reaching out could create a domino effect—inspiring your friends and family to confide in you or someone else about their own life challenges.

No One Will Understand You

People with almost anorexia often worry that loved ones will not understand their pain. While it's true that others may not fully appreciate the "why" behind almost anorexia, they can still be an important source of support. When Jenni told her family and friends that she felt fat, she needed people to acknowledge her distress, not argue about her real or imagined weight fluctuations. It felt very supportive, for instance, when her mom responded, "I believe that you feel that way, and I am sorry. I don't understand why you feel fat, but I'm still here for you." That said, you know your loved ones best. If there's a history of dysfunctional behavior (such as emotional, sexual, or physical abuse), then consider reaching out to alternative supports like another family member, friend, or health care professional.

I'm Supposed to Be a Role Model

If you are a caregiver whom others view as a role model, you may feel intense pressure to be the paragon of health. Dr. Thomas has worked with many mothers, doctors, and therapists who have felt compelled to keep their almost anorexia hidden. In particular, women with bulimic symptoms often feel they must lead a "double life"[7]—projecting a veneer of confidence and competence in public, but bingeing and purging in private. Not only is this daily performance emotionally draining and physically exhausting, but keeping your disordered eating a secret will only exacerbate your feelings of fraudulence. Although recovering from almost anorexia may require acknowledging your imperfections, it will ultimately improve your ability to model healthy behaviors to others. Follow the example of former United Kingdom Deputy Prime Minister John Prescott who spoke out about his fight with bulimia while still a member of Parliament. Referring to why he hid his illness for ten years, sixty-nine-year-old Prescott told the British Broadcasting Corporation, "I never admitted to this out of the shame and embarrassment. I found it difficult as a man like me to admit that I suffered from bulimia."[8] But today, Lord Prescott's journey of healing has inspired countless men to improve their relationship with food.

My Symptoms Are Not Really That Bad

Individuals with almost anorexia and other officially recognized eating disorders often feel that their eating problems are not serious enough to warrant treatment.[9] Many feel unworthy of help. Some may even feel like they have not "mastered" the eating disorder the way they had wanted. We hope that by the time you have reached this point in the book, you understand that almost anorexia is extremely serious and that seeking help now is the best way to prevent your disordered eating from getting worse. All who suffer both need and deserve help.

Jenni's Journey

For years, Ed told me, "Sure, you are different with food, but you don't have a real problem." When I finally realized that he was lying and that I did, in fact, struggle with an eating disorder, I thought that I could get better on my own by reading self-help books. But it didn't take long before I learned that, although books provide hope and guidance, they alone can't fix you. Because I lived across the country from my family at the time, I decided to tell my then-boyfriend about what was going on. I was so ashamed of my secret that I couldn't even speak to him face to face. Instead, I tucked a pamphlet about eating disorders under my couch pillow in the living room while I hid under the covers on my bed in the bedroom. Luckily, he knew what I was trying to say. (Today, I am a lot better at direct communication!) We decided to call my parents, who responded with complete love and support. They were also surprised. While they had noticed my weight loss in college, the doctor had given me a clean bill of health, so they had thought I was okay. At first, I asked my parents to keep Ed a secret. But we soon realized that

CONTINUED ON NEXT PAGE

CONTINUED FROM PREVIOUS PAGE

we all needed support from additional family and friends. My dad said, "If you had cancer, we wouldn't keep it a secret. You have a life-threatening illness. It is nothing to be embarrassed about." So, slowly, I shared my story with others and sought out much-needed support. Back then—hiding under the covers—I never would have guessed I'd write a book about my journey. Maybe you can't imagine telling someone in your life. But just because you can't imagine it doesn't mean it can't happen. After all, you are reading one of my books right now.

Tell Someone

Telling someone about your disordered eating is essential. In Dr. Thomas's study of young adults who attended the college-based National Eating Disorder Screening Program, 98 percent of those who were concerned about their own eating or weight had disclosed these worries to someone. Keep in mind that these individuals were willing participants in a screening program, so most had already taken the first step of telling someone like a friend (87 percent), partner (57 percent), or parent (53 percent). Less than half (46 percent) had disclosed their concerns to a health care professional—but those who did were significantly more likely to have sought treatment two years later.[10] We know that reaching out might be intensely frightening. The fear of being rejected can feel intolerable, especially if you already struggle with social anxiety. So, how can you actually do it?

We recommend connecting face to face with a person you trust. This might be a friend, family member, teacher, or doctor.

Let the person know in advance that you need to discuss something important. Make arrangements to talk at a specific time and place so that you will not be interrupted. Speak from your heart and be honest. If the thought of speaking out loud about your difficulty with food paralyzes you, consider writing a letter or email instead and then giving this to the person. Try to be present when your words are read. But if, similar to Jenni's experience, you cannot imagine being in the same space with someone when you ask for help, walk into a different room or simply send the note. A letter can be one step toward a face-to-face talk or even an introduction to an in-person discussion—when you are ready. Do the best that you can; there is no perfect way. The only thing that truly matters is that you reach out.

Share this book with friends and family members if you have found it helpful. You may even want to highlight certain sections that feel especially relevant for you. Several of Dr. Thomas's patients have brought highlighted copies of Jenni's books to therapy sessions. Others have put stickers on passages that they want their partner or parents to read. In this way, the second person reading gains not only the book's knowledge but also unique insights into how you yourself are feeling.

Get creative and do what works for you. Chad was surprised to learn how much support was available when he finally sought it out.

Chad

"No, I can't do breakfast this morning. I need to get to school early to study," Chad called to his parents as he scurried out of the house—the one where he had grown up and still chose to live in order to save money. During his drive to medical school,

Chad sipped black coffee and listened to a recording he had made of himself reading a biochemistry textbook. While he knew that some would consider this overstudying, the compulsion to do whatever it took to keep his string of A's going was just too strong to overcome. Lately, he had lacked energy and school seemed more difficult.

Parking in a remote campus lot, he began his morning hike to class. Chad claimed to like the distant lot because there was less chance of his parents' car getting hit or scratched by reckless undergraduates, but the truth was that he felt relief in the long walk. With his rigorous study schedule, he just didn't have time to hit the gym. And he couldn't imagine going through even a single day without some form of exercise.

Nearing the gross anatomy lab, Chad smiled when he saw Cassie. She was the one student on campus with whom he had regular conversations—and that was only because she had been assigned as his student mentor during orientation. Aside from Cassie and his parents, Chad didn't connect with many people. (He knew that his 302 Facebook friends didn't count, since he rarely interacted with them, even online.) Noting his heavy backpack, Cassie joked, "Are you ever going to replace that dinosaur laptop?" With that, she easily slipped her ultrathin tablet into her handbag and said, "This is so much easier to carry. Plus, it was actually made this century!" Chad laughed; this was a running joke between them. He didn't mind his super-slow, not to mention truly heavy, computer. He saved money by keeping his laptop as long as possible. Plus, he thought, *The extra weight helps me to burn more calories.* They made plans to have lunch together and went their separate ways to class.

Others found it hard to believe that Chad wasn't dating Cassie, but he surely wasn't interested—not in that way. From age thirteen, he knew that he liked men, although he hadn't revealed this to anyone. He was pretty sure it wouldn't go over very well in his conservative hometown. *Besides, I can date later,* he thought. Delaying gratification came easy to him.

After a long morning in lab, he was ready for his lunch break—but not necessarily to eat. Chad just enjoyed escaping the pressure cooker of his overly competitive classmates and looked forward to walking alone outside. Keeping his gaze close to the ground to avoid having to talk with anyone, he walked briskly to meet Cassie, who greeted him at the door holding a slice of pizza and a side salad. "I'll save you a spot while you get something to eat," she offered. "No," Chad said, "I'm not hungry. I ate a snack earlier." Chad carried granola bars and apples around with him—another reason his backpack was so heavy. He didn't trust the dining hall food, not knowing exactly what ingredients were in each item. Cassie chose not to push him about eating, as it never seemed to help. Still, she couldn't help but notice how pale and gaunt he had become since the beginning of the semester.

Before rushing off to class, she decided that if she couldn't tell Chad yet again that she was concerned about his eating, she could at least express her feelings indirectly. "Here," she said, handing him a pamphlet about the National Eating Disorders Screening Program (NEDSP) that was currently being held on campus. She fumbled with her words, "You'll be having that eating disorder lecture soon in . . . um . . . one of your classes. You might want to talk with these people for some insider information. Maybe you can get ahead!"

Chad knew a little about eating disorders and had even wondered about his own behavior. After realizing that he needed a belt to hold up the pants his mom had bought him just a few months earlier, he had looked up anorexia nervosa in his textbook. He learned that he had not lost enough weight to receive an official diagnosis, which he found reassuring: *I'm not that bad.* Plus, as a future doctor, he couldn't admit to having a mental health problem—even if he did.

Leaving the dining hall, Chad saw the NEDSP table set up just outside. *Maybe Cassie is right*, he thought. A friendly woman greeted him and explained how the screening process worked, so he decided to take the simple test to get an inside look at the questions someone with an actual eating disorder might be asked. As he marked his answers, Chad began to suspect that he might, in fact, have a problem. ("Are you terrified of gaining weight?" *Usually.* "Do you find yourself preoccupied with food?" *Always.* "Do you avoid food with high-carbohydrate content?" *Often.*) Sure enough, the results recommended that he see a health professional for a complete evaluation. Always eager to follow the rules and do the right thing, he made an appointment with a school counselor for the very next day.

Your Social Network

During his descent into almost anorexia, specifically atypical anorexia, Chad did not know many people who could have thrown him a lifeline. Do you? In collaboration with clinical psychologist Michael E. Berrett, we have developed the tool in figure 9 for assessing your current level of social support. The pie-shaped sections represent various arenas of your life: family, friends, colleagues or classmates, treatment relationships, spiritual groups, and other relationships (such as teammates or neighbors). Within each arena, your relationships will vary in closeness—represented by increasingly smaller concentric circles. A "casual" relationship might be one that you have with a classmate or colleague. Even though you see this person on a regular basis at work or school, you don't really connect on an emotional level. Acquaintances fit into this category. "Close" people in your life are those with whom you share some emotional intimacy. You choose to spend time with them. Your "closest" relationships are the ones in which you are deeply open with your innermost thoughts and feelings. You interact with these people often and feel you can truly trust them to help you through difficult times.

In each arena of life, who gives you support? Visualize in figure 9 how Chad would answer this question. Then, within the different sections of figure 10, write the names of those who belong in that area, or draw concentric circles in a notebook and write down the names. You might notice that you have a lot of opportunity to increase connectedness—like Chad did. Specifically, while Cassie is a "close" friend with whom he spends a lot of time, he hasn't yet shared with her the most important struggles he is currently facing—his sexual orientation and disordered eating. Similarly, while Chad interacts casually with his fellow med students and Facebook friends, he doesn't connect with any of them on an emotional level. There are some other arenas in which Chad does not have anyone listed, including other relationships, such as teams or clubs, and spiritual groups or leaders. While spirituality might include specific religious beliefs, it can also be connected to mindfulness, music, nature, service, principled living, and more. Go inward and determine what spirituality means to you. Dr. Berrett, coauthor of *Spiritual Approaches in the Treatment of Women with Eating Disorders*,[11] has said that "spirituality is like Tabasco sauce—just a little can have a big kick in recovery."[12] Indeed, there is evidence that interventions designed to enrich spirituality may improve the effectiveness of standard eating disorder treatment.[13] As you review your own social network, do you see any opportunities to increase support? Do you have "casual" relationships that could become "close"? Are there any arenas (like "other") that are currently empty but could be filled? Remember that quality is more important than quantity.

Figure 9.
Chad's Social Support Network

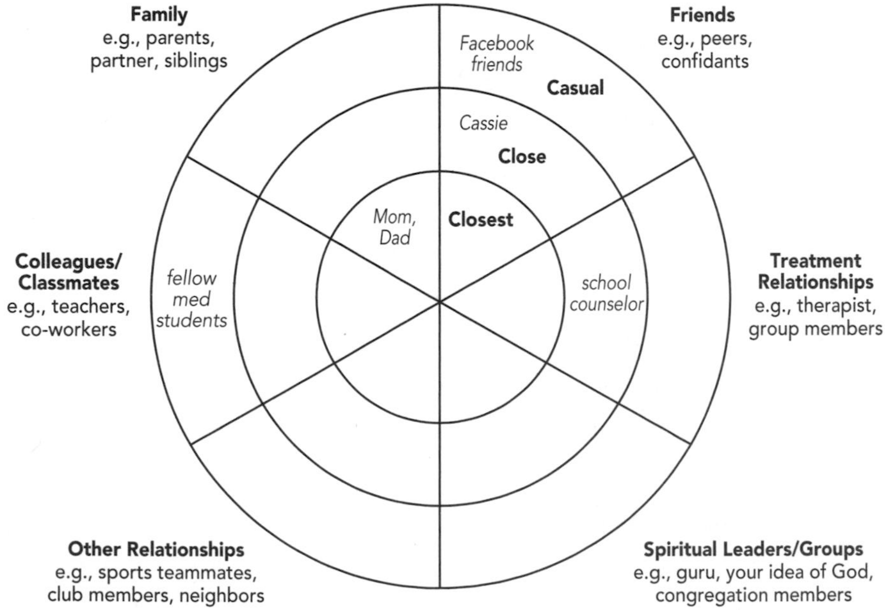

Figure 10.

Your Social Support Network

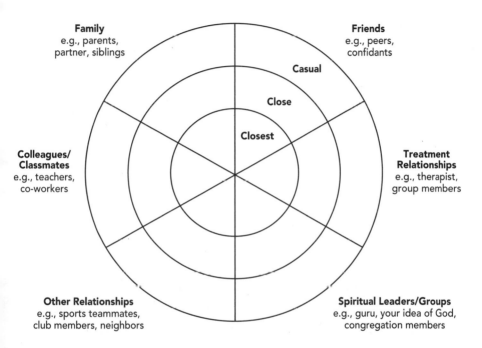

Family
e.g., parents,
partner, siblings

Friends
e.g., peers,
confidants

Casual

Close

Closest

**Colleagues/
Classmates**
e.g., teachers,
co-workers

**Treatment
Relationships**
e.g., therapist,
group members

Other Relationships
e.g., sports teammates,
club members, neighbors

Spiritual Leaders/Groups
e.g., guru, your idea of God,
congregation members

Adapted from M.E. Berrett's *"Reciprocal Social Support of Adolescents: An Assessment Model and Measure,"* 1985[14]

This exercise can be downloaded at www.almostanorexic.com.

Focus on surrounding yourself with people who specifically support your recovery. This often means teaching others how to help you. What do they do and say that's helpful or unhelpful? Tell them. If you notice that certain people in your life are always on diets, ask them not to talk about their weight-loss plans around you. Change the conversation. When others are not responsive to your needs, you may need to distance yourself for a while or even permanently. And this goes for online relationships too. On Facebook, "hide" posts from people who constantly comment negatively about food and body image, and don't hesitate to delete a "friend" or decline a "friend request" (stay completely away from a person in cyberspace). Peer influence is powerful and may even be long lasting. In one study, women whose college roommates dieted more frequently had a greater drive for thinness and were more likely to report purging a full ten years later—long after they had moved off campus and started their adult lives.[15] Social support is important, yet that support needs to be the right kind from the right people.

Friend Requests

In addition to real-life connections, technology enables most of us to relate in cyberspace. Harness the power of the Internet to build your support team. You might want to reach out online to pro-recovery sites like www.mentorconnect-ed.org, Mentor-CONNECT, where you can find a peer recovery mentor for free. Visit Jenni's author Facebook page at www.facebook.com/LifeWithoutEd to join positive discussions with others about recovery from disordered eating. Connect with people who are fully recovered. Follow people on Twitter who tweet inspirational quotes and sayings; avoid those who promote pro-ana ideas. Use technology to your advantage. Text messaging and email can be particularly helpful in keeping yourself accountable. Send a message to someone at each meal, or Instagram a photo of a challenge item to seek support from a friend. Turn your mobile phone into a recovery tool by programming names and numbers of key players on your support team. The support you need can literally be at your fingertips.

Although linking with people on social media sites is relatively easy, this is not always the case in real life. In the real world, you can't just click a button to send a friend request, "follow" a certain person, or even "like" someone. Internet friends can be helpful and supportive, but they should not be your sole way to stay connected. So, how can you get connected in person? If you are still in school, your varying class schedule will provide you with a fresh opportunity to meet people. Make an attempt to sit by new people, smile, and say hello. Be an active member of school clubs rather than just adding another group to your résumé. Start a group of your own.

Being out of school makes it more challenging to meet people, especially if you work from home as a stay-at-home parent or as a self-employed individual. But it is still possible. Except when she receives special deliveries at her door, Jenni does not run into many people when she writes in her home—where she works alone. To meet others, she sometimes totes her laptop to coffee shops. Here are some other ideas:

- Rather than always waiting for invitations, reach out to people you already know. Invite someone to watch a movie or share a meal. You might end up becoming closer with someone you've known for years.

241

- Meet others by volunteering, joining an intramural sports team, or participating in activities with those who have a similar faith.

- Visit www.meetup.com to learn about people in your area who share common interests. You will find groups that focus on varied interests, including knitting, crocheting, playing board or video games, and traveling. There are also groups that come together for sports, parenting, writing, photography, and more.

- If your Facebook friends really are people who mean a lot to you, then make a point to socialize in person—not just in cyberspace.

• • •

Don't be discouraged if things don't work out at first. Keep trying. When you do spend time with trusted others who truly matter to you, then push yourself to discuss more real and meaningful topics, such as feelings, ideas, concerns, hopes, desires, and dreams. When you feel close to people, be vulnerable by opening up about what really matters to you rather than just talking about the weather or the latest clothing styles. Although there is nothing inherently wrong with discussing the weather, relationships can offer much more. For example, Dr. Thomas loves clothes, but she talks to her girlfriends about much more than handbags and shoes. Strive for quality over quantity.

Chad's Friend Requests

"You are extremely isolated, Chad," the counselor said at the end of their first appointment. "To improve your relationship with food, one of your priorities will be to get connected with others." Chad groaned inwardly. He had always done almost everything alone—and quite successfully—so he didn't believe that recovering from almost anorexia would be any different. *But I guess I am feeling a bit lonely,* he thought to himself. After Cassie responded to Chad's disclosure in a heartfelt way and even connected him with another student in recovery from an eating disorder, he slowly gained the strength to reach out to even more people, including his parents, who were compassionate and eager to help. Although Chad didn't reveal his eating problems to everyone, he started to build a network of people around him. He even joined—albeit secretly—the gay, lesbian, bisexual, and transgender student organization on campus and surprisingly discovered that a couple of others in the group struggled with disordered eating. Not long after, he started inviting his classmates over to his house for marathon study sessions—with pizza. He was eating his favorite food again. Slowly, Chad's relationships were taking the place of almost anorexia.

Adding Professional Support

Recovering from disordered eating might be compared to completing a jigsaw puzzle. Many pieces must come together for healing to take place. For some, professional help is a vital piece of the puzzle. How do you know if you or your loved one needs additional support? As we mentioned in chapter 1, anyone who scores in the unhealthy range on the EAT-26 should absolutely seek a professional evaluation. If you scored in the healthy range but are nonetheless suffering intensely due to your relationship with food and weight, we suggest that you consider getting an evaluation as well. Effective treatments for disordered eating are available. Although most people with almost anorexia and other officially recognized eating disorders will benefit from outpatient psychotherapy, medical care is critical, adjunctive medication can be useful, and as mentioned previously, dietary counseling is very helpful. Sometimes, hospitalization is necessary.

Individual Psychotherapy

Cognitive-behavioral therapy (CBT) is the best studied and best established treatment for bulimia nervosa, binge eating disorder, and EDNOS.[16] CBT is a skills-based treatment that focuses on modifying cognitions (e.g., harmful beliefs about eating, shape, and weight) and behaviors (e.g., dietary rules, binge eating, or purging). Many of the techniques described in this book draw from a CBT approach, including normalizing eating, developing alternatives to bingeing and purging, reducing body checking, and preventing relapse. Interestingly, the "do the next right thing" concept that helped Jenni so much during her recovery is an important part of the CBT approach—and she didn't even know it at the time! There is also evidence that other types of individual psychotherapy are effective in the treatment of eating disorders, such as specialist supportive clinical management, psychodynamic therapy, interpersonal therapy, dialectical behavioral therapy, and acceptance and commitment therapy.

Dietary Counseling

An important player on an eating disorder treatment team can be a registered dietitian who specializes in the illness. Often, a dietitian will initially work with someone to simply eat more regularly throughout the day, possibly using a food plan or some other form of structure. Ultimately, a dietitian can guide an individual to become more flexible with food and to achieve intuitive eating. Family members can also learn important strategies to support their loved one during mealtimes.

Family Treatment

Other effective therapies for almost anorexia enlist the support of loved ones. One key evidence-based approach is family-based treatment (FBT) for children and adolescents with anorexia. In FBT, parents are encouraged to correct their child's malnutrition by providing a structured and energy-rich meal plan. After steady weight gain has been established, food choices are gradually returned to the child, and family members are invited to explore the ways in which the eating disorder has affected family dynamics and to orchestrate a smooth return to normal adolescent development.[17] The concept of separating the individual from the eating disorder—which Jenni popularized in her book *Life Without Ed*—is a central tenet of FBT. Uniting Couples in the Treatment of Anorexia Nervosa is a related approach that enlists the support of a partner to assist an adult in overcoming anorexia.[18] No matter which therapeutic family approach is utilized, the important thing is that, in the vast majority of cases, families want to be involved in treatment and can learn to provide great support when included in recovery efforts.

Medication

The U.S. Food and Drug Administration (FDA) has not approved any medication specifically for the treatment of anorexia nervosa. Furthermore, the FDA cannot do so for almost anorexia, since it is not an officially recognized eating disorder.

Because of this, drugs used as adjuncts to psychotherapy for subclinical eating disorders are always considered off-label. Fluoxetine (Prozac) has been shown to reduce binge/purge frequency in bulimia nervosa and is FDA-approved for this indication.[19] There is also some evidence that olanzapine (Zyprexa) may facilitate weight gain and reduce obsessive symptoms in anorexia nervosa.[20] Among obese individuals with binge eating disorder, topiramate (Topamax) has been shown to reduce binge frequency and facilitate weight loss.[21] These are the most common medications in use as of this writing, but as more research is done, they may be supplemented or replaced by others. Your health care professional is the best source of current information about which medications are appropriate for you. Notably, certain medications are contraindicated for the treatment of eating disorders. Specifically, bupropion (Wellbutrin) was associated with an increased rate of seizures in one study of women with bulimia nervosa,[22] and monoamine oxidase inhibitors (a class of antidepressant medications) require adherence to a highly restricted diet that may interfere with eating disorder treatment goals.

Early in her treatment, Jenni refused all medications, telling her doctors that she wanted to recover "on her own." She thought taking medicine would make her "weak." But she ultimately realized that it was no great achievement to continue suffering when she could have been feeling better. She doesn't need them anymore, but she's glad that she had the strength to ask for them when she did. If you believe that medication might be helpful for you, consult with a doctor who has experience in treating patients with eating disorders. And remember, medication cannot take the place of—and always works best with— proper nourishment.

Hospitalization

Some individuals with almost anorexia and eating disorders are not able to beat Ed in outpatient treatment while living at home. In these severe cases, more intensive treatment options include day treatment, residential care, or inpatient hospitalization. How do you know if you need to seek a higher level of care for disordered eating? Key signs that inpatient hospitalization is needed include very low body weight or rapid weight loss, medical complications, suicidal thoughts, escalating or severe symptoms (such as an inability to eat independently or frequent purging throughout the entire day), and/or complete lack of benefit from outpatient care.[23] If you think you or a loved one might need to be hospitalized for almost anorexia, speak with your clinician immediately or go to your nearest emergency room for a professional evaluation.

• • •

Depending on the treatment approach, you might need different types of professionals to help you. Many people call the group of professionals who help them a "treatment team." Your treatment team might include a therapist, psychiatrist, primary care physician, dietitian, other medical specialists, or any combination of these. You might decide to join a peer support group and/or a group led by a therapist. Although no randomized controlled study has ever investigated the effectiveness of Twelve Step groups for eating disorders,[24] some people have found Eating Disorders Anonymous (which does *not* require abstinence from specific foods) to be helpful. See appendix C for ideas on assembling a treatment team, finding a group, paying for care, and identifying a therapist who specializes in eating disorders and who is right for you.

How to Help Someone Else

One of the best ways to find out how to help a loved one with almost anorexia is to ask, "How can I support you?" People who are struggling must teach those around them what feels supportive and what doesn't. Different strategies work best for different people. Modeling healthy attitudes and behaviors with food and body image is, of course, always helpful. Talk positively about your body. Bragging about your diet or lamenting over how much you overate is not supportive. Don't discuss food in terms of "good" and "bad." Talking about important topics beyond calories, food, and dieting not only can be helpful but also can nurture and strengthen your relationship.

Throughout the recovery process, never forget about your own life and needs. This includes sometimes taking time off from being the supporter and getting help for yourself. Hang out with a friend to talk about something not related to Ed. Or consider joining the National Eating Disorders Association (NEDA) Parent, Family & Friends Network, which is open to people around the globe. In fact, as a part of this program, bilingual NEDA navigators are available to guide you to resources.

You may have heard that your loved ones won't get better unless they are doing it for themselves. We completely disagree with this line of thought. If your loved one lacks the personal desire to get better, you can certainly encourage him or her to do it for any other greater purpose or cause. For example, some will want to get better for the people they love. In the beginning, it doesn't matter why someone is getting help—to make someone else happy, to go back to college, or for another reason. All that matters is that they are getting support. People often start off getting better "for a loved one," but after they are no longer malnourished and can think more clearly, they end up doing it for themselves as well. We have provided a list of do's and don'ts for loved ones in table 14. For further reading, we recommend the book *Skills-Based Learning for Caring for a Loved One with an Eating Disorder: The New Maudsley Method.*[25]

· · ·

Eating disorders tear relationships apart, but recovery brings people together. In her memoir of anorexia recovery, *Beating Ana*, Shannon Cutts theorized, "Relationships replace eating disorders. Period. The End."[26] We agree. Through the healing process, you and your loved ones can become closer than ever. Relationships play a vital role in reaching a full recovery.

Table 14.

Do's and Don'ts of Supporting a Loved One Who Has Almost Anorexia

Don't	Do
1. Blame yourself for your loved one's eating problem	1. Educate yourself about eating disorders; appreciate that the symptoms are not a product of willfulness
2. Simply ignore the eating problem and hope it goes away on its own	2. Express your concern and ask your loved one how you can be helpful
3. Be hostile, critical, or bullying; this will only give your loved one opportunities to practice arguments for not changing	3. Be warm, firm, and direct; ask your loved one if he or she has his or her own reasons for wanting to change
4. Collude with the eating disorder (such as preparing "diet" meals or taking over responsibilities for your loved one, which will only reinforce the illness)	4. Encourage your loved one to seek professional help if needed, and attend sessions if invited by your loved one's clinician
5. Try to talk your loved one out of eating disorder beliefs by using logic, or beat yourself up for not completely understanding his or her struggle	5. Let your loved one know that you believe that he or she feels fat or is worried about having eaten too much, but that you yourself do not agree
6. Provide constant reassurance around food and weight (for example, "Yes, it's okay to eat that much," "No, you aren't fat"); this is a battle you cannot win	6. Gently let your loved one know that it is unhelpful to get into arguments about weight or shape; then try changing the subject instead
7. Forget about your own self-care; you need to care for yourself in order to retain the calmness and compassion necessary to care for your loved one	7. Get support for yourself, including professional help, if necessary; model healthy eating and self-esteem by avoiding unhealthy dieting and fat talk

This exercise can be downloaded at www.almostanorexic.com.

| 11 |

Don't Settle for Almost Recovered

Full freedom from almost anorexia is possible. Don't let anyone convince you otherwise—especially Ed, who may find this chapter too hopeful. Both research and clinical experience support the reality that people who struggle with food and body image problems can ultimately reach a place we call fully recovered. This means a lot more than just learning how to eat normally and restoring your weight. Recovery also means getting your life back. It took time, but Samantha, who battled almost anorexia on her way out of anorexia nervosa, did just that.

Samantha

Dr. Thomas first met Samantha during her post-doctoral fellowship, when she got paged to do a consult in the hospital's psychiatric inpatient unit. Noting the "trainee" designation on Dr. Thomas's badge, Samantha immediately sat up in bed and remarked, "I'll be a great training case for you. I probably have the worst case of anorexia you'll ever see."

As Samantha told her story, waving her stick-thin arms for emphasis, Dr. Thomas realized that Samantha might not be kidding. At twenty-one years old, she had struggled with anorexia for ten years, racking up admissions at every single inpatient and residential treatment center in New England. "They keep kicking me out because they don't know what to do with me," she boasted. "I've even ripped out my feeding tube and jumped out of first-floor windows to avoid eating meals. Most doctors are scared to work with me." With Samantha's frighteningly frail body and a history of a dangerously low heart rate and hypokalemia (lower than normal level of potassium in the bloodstream), Dr. Thomas could see why. Before being admitted, Samantha was bingeing and purging up to seven times per day. On nonbinge days, she fasted completely.

But as Samantha continued talking, Dr. Thomas thought she detected a hairline crack in Samantha's brave facade. The truth was that Samantha had given up a lot to maintain her anorexia. Her parents had stopped contacting her after they'd lost their petition for medical guardianship, and she was currently in a relationship with a man who physically abused her. After riding a merry-go-round of eating disorder remissions and relapses, Samantha felt exhausted and hopeless. "I don't know what they're teaching you here," she said, rolling her eyes. "But you should know that eating disorders are something you never really get over." Dr. Thomas cocked her head for a minute and replied conspiratorially, "A lot of people think that, but since I'm still in training, I'm not so sure. How would you like to prove them wrong?"

It took four years of therapy and several more inpatient stays, but Samantha finally beat anorexia. She worked incredibly hard to get her weight up to the bottom of the normal range for her body. Although she still restricted some and binged and purged intermittently, her disordered-eating behaviors were far less frequent and intense than before. She ultimately broke up with her abusive boyfriend and started dating a man named Eric, whose steadfast calmness was the perfect foil for her dramatic flair. After they got married in a small ceremony with family and close friends, Samantha was thrilled to learn she was pregnant. She resolved to stop bingeing and purging completely and to markedly increase her calorie intake to support the baby's growth. She couldn't have been happier when she gave birth to Madison, a healthy baby girl. Samantha was so pleased with how far she had progressed that she didn't believe she needed to go any further. So when Dr. Thomas suggested that she bring a chocolate bar to eat at their first postnatal therapy session, Samantha snapped. "What do you want from me?" she demanded. "I've gained weight. I've stopped bingeing and purging. I even had a baby! Why do I have to prove that I can eat some stupid chocolate bar now—when I've already done everything you've asked?"

Dr. Thomas validated Samantha's extremely hard work but then expressed her concern that, although Samantha had overcome anorexia nervosa, she continued to struggle with almost anorexia, or residual symptoms of her eating disorder. For example, Samantha ate the same three "safe" meals every day and brought her own food in plastic containers when she visited family for the holidays. Sleep deprived from waking up multiple times per night to nurse her infant, she still prepared three dinners every night—a salad for herself, organic baby food for Madison, and meat and potatoes for her husband.

While her baby napped, she felt compelled to do postnatal yoga DVDs or hit the elliptical machine. She obsessed about losing the "baby weight." Although she did lose this weight, she never lost enough to be diagnosed with anorexia again. However, she suffered from atypical anorexia at this point in her life, a time when she didn't even allow her friends to throw her a baby shower: she didn't want them to take photos of her "looking fat."

"You have come further than you ever thought you could, but I know you can have an even healthier relationship with food," Dr. Thomas persisted. "Do you really want to settle for almost recovered?"

How Free Do You Want to Be?

During the recovery process from either almost anorexia or a full-blown eating disorder, you may notice that you reach certain plateaus. Maybe you finally stop bingeing, which is a triumph, but you are restricting more than ever—a problem that many people don't like to admit. Or possibly you finally are eating enough, but now you experience intense feelings of fatness. During these times, it is crucial to pat yourself on the back and acknowledge how far you have come. But it is equally important to recognize that you still have some room to grow. In a longitudinal study conducted by clinical psychologist Kamryn Eddy and colleagues, many women with an intake diagnosis of anorexia or bulimia nervosa recovered during the nine-year follow-up period. However, the transition was rarely black-and-white; more than three quarters exhibited subclinical eating disorders at some point during the study.[1]

The question ultimately becomes "How free do you want to

be?" You don't have to settle for lingering eating-disordered thoughts and attitudes. With time, patience, and continued growth, you can ultimately reach a place where you don't even hear Ed anymore. Jenni often compares her personal Ed to a muscle: When she engaged Ed and obeyed him, he grew bigger and stronger. But when she stopped listening and began to trust herself, Ed atrophied like a muscle that wasn't getting used. Essentially, her eating disorder wasted away slowly, just like her calf muscle had when she broke her foot.

When Jenni's eating disorder "muscle" was atrophying, it wasn't uncommon for a conversation with Ed to sound something like this:

Ed: You need to lose a few pounds.

Jenni:

Ed: Let's go to the store and binge like old times.

Jenni:

Ed: Earth to Jenni—are you still there?

Yes, you got it: these were not really conversations at all. Eventually, Jenni reached a point where she simply ignored Ed. The more she was able to do this, the less he spoke. In time, he stopped talking altogether.

When your disordered-eating behaviors and thoughts first fade into the background, you might find yourself maintaining a healthy weight and even a positive body image—and yet, feel completely miserable. Once again, this is just a phase. It indicates that you have made tremendous progress. It means keep going. The beginning of a life without Ed can feel unfamiliar. Feelings of depression can even arise when you stop turning to (or away from) food. (If the depressive symptoms persist, and especially if they get worse, we recommend consulting a health care professional for assessment and treatment. Even a mild depression can undermine your success in becoming fully recovered from almost anorexia or other eating disorders.) But you will ultimately find joy and peace if you face your fears both at the table and on the scale. A full recovery, of course, does not mean that you will be free from all problems in your life. (If we figure out how to do that, we will definitely write another book!) While people can recover from almost anorexia and other officially recognized eating disorders, no one is ever completely recovered from life, which will always be a journey with diverse challenges. But when you are recovered, you will have the strength—more than ever before—to face obstacles head-on while simultaneously knowing when it's okay to let go. Because life is a continual growth process, some people, especially those who participate in Twelve Step programs, refer to themselves as being "in recovery." But try not to get caught up in semantics. The important thing to know is that independence from disordered eating is possible, regardless of what you personally choose to call it.

What does freedom mean to you? In her book *100 Questions & Answers about Eating Disorders*, marriage and family therapist Carolyn Costin, who herself recovered from anorexia nervosa, defines recovery this way: "Being recovered is when a person can accept his or her natural body size and shape and no longer has a self-destructive relationship with food or exercise. When you are recovered, food and weight take a proper perspective in your life, and what you weigh is not more important than who you are; in fact, actual numbers are of little or no importance at all. When recovered, you will not compromise your health or betray your soul to look a certain way, wear a certain size, or reach a certain number on a scale. When you are recovered, you do not use eating disorder behaviors to deal with, distract from, or cope with other problems."[2] Are you settling for barely recovered? To help you find out, see the table 15 checklist. Similar to the normal eating table in chapter 7, you might find yourself in both columns at any given point on the same day. The goal is to move, in all areas listed, more toward "fully recovered" on the right. And, ultimately, if you keep moving, you will find yourself living fully recovered.

If You Don't Believe Us . . .

You may believe that once you struggle with disordered eating, you always will. A study of individuals previously treated for anorexia nervosa found that 25 percent did not believe that full recovery was possible.[3] At the height of her illness, Jenni was among them. But she ultimately broke free—after hearing Ed's voice for more than twenty years. Similarly, Dr. Thomas recently worked with a remarkable woman who made major improvements at the age of sixty-five—after fifty years of anorexia!

But if you don't believe us, believe the research. In three recent studies of individuals with EDNOS who received out-patient therapy for eating disorders (some after having been ill for many years), two-thirds were abstinent from disordered-eating behaviors one year after completing treatment.[4] And although treatment typically speeds the recovery process, two recent prospective studies demonstrated that more than three-quarters of those with EDNOS recovered over the course of

Table 15.

Recovered. (Period.)

Are you settling for a mediocre version of recovery from almost anorexia?

What barely recovered looks like	What fully recovered looks like
1. Your eating-disordered behaviors are causing you to maintain an unhealthy weight for your body (for example, your weight is slightly below or just within normal range—despite professionals encouraging you to gain more).	1. You accept the weight your body naturally maintains when you are no longer engaging in eating-disordered behaviors.
2. Shifts in weight make you very uncomfortable. You do your best to avoid them.	2. You are able to tolerate natural shifts in weight that accompany worthwhile activities (such as pregnancy, vacation, and aging).
3. You restrict "just a little." You binge and purge on occasion—but only to get yourself through tough times.	3. You never use eating-disordered behaviors like restricting, bingeing, or purging. They are not on your list of coping skills.
4. Thoughts about food and weight occupy a large amount of time, disrupting your life.	4. Thoughts about food and weight do not occupy a great deal of your time. Instead, you focus your energy on truly living.
5. You tolerate your body. You loathe imperfections.	5. You love your body. You accept imperfections.
6. Your primary focus regarding your body is appearance.	6. You appreciate your body for what it does rather than focusing exclusively on what it looks like.
7. You exercise almost solely to maintain your weight. You "have to" exercise and don't enjoy it much.	7. You exercise intuitively for health and fun. You give your body enough rest too.
8. Personality traits that contributed to the development of your eating disorder (such as perfectionism, impulsivity, and obsessive-compulsiveness) cause problems in other life domains.	8. You channel your unique personality traits in pursuit of important life goals. Perfectionism becomes the pursuit of excellence, impulsivity becomes spontaneity, and obsessive-compulsiveness becomes conscientiousness.

This exercise can be downloaded at www.almostanorexic.com.

four to five years, regardless of whether they were treated during the course of the study.[5] And we continue to be hopeful about the rest.

There are many scientific reasons to predict that recovery rates for almost anorexia and other eating disorders will continue to improve with time. First, many recovery statistics are based on individuals who were ill long before effective treatments were developed. Indeed, therapist manuals for the two best-studied outpatient eating disorder treatments—family-based treatment for anorexia and cognitive-behavioral therapy for bulimia and EDNOS—were just published in the last few years.[6] This means that true recovery rates today may be even higher than earlier studies reflect. Second, novel treatments are constantly being developed, and clinical researchers are increasingly raising the bar for testing them. Whereas previous studies

Jenni's Journey

One of the first clinicians I ever told about my problems with food said, "Your eating disorder is like diabetes. You might learn to manage it, but it will always be in the back of your mind." Apparently, I was doomed for a lifelong battle with food—a substance that I was going to have to see at least three times a day, every single day, for the rest of my life. There was absolutely no hope in that message—I felt overwhelmed. If I had ultimately believed this perspective, I might have settled for various partial versions of recovery, including a time when I ate the same exact food for breakfast and lunch each day, or a period when I had just accepted that I was going to hate my body forever. Or I might have remained in that place where my eating-disordered behaviors had stopped but I lived in a state of worry

CONTINUED ON NEXT PAGE

CONTINUED FROM PREVIOUS PAGE

and unhappiness—feeling a sense of impending doom—most of the time. But instead of putting my faith in "mediocre," I stopped seeing that clinician and surrounded myself with people —professionals, family members, and friends—who had faith that I could fully recover. I chose to believe that I could get completely better, too, and I finally did. Today, I eat what I'm truly hungry for at mealtimes, I accept and love my body, and I'm finally happy. This doesn't mean that I wake up every morning with a smile plastered on my face, but rather that I feel a deep sense of contentment even during difficult times. When I have trouble finding this inner joy, I turn to gratitude, which always helps. I don't turn to food. Sometimes, I still worry too much (especially about dating!), but again I know how to calm my fears without overeating or restricting. Hope in a full recovery has made all of the difference.

required just weight gain and menstrual recovery to declare anorexia treatment successful,[7] recent studies (including some of those described earlier) have used more rigorous definitions of recovery that also require abstinence from eating-disordered behaviors and normalization of attitudes toward food and weight.[8]

Fall Down Seven Times, Stand Up Eight

Before Dr. Thomas became Dr. Thomas, she was an aspiring ballerina at the Anaheim Ballet. Her teachers had a tradition that whenever a student—whether beginning or advanced—fell down, the whole class would clap and shout "Progress!" They believed that dancers who executed every step perfectly couldn't be truly challenging themselves and that real improvement could only come from falling down, getting back up, and trying again. Given how many of their students went on to dance professionally (Dr. Thomas's childhood rival, Amy Watson, is now a principal dancer with the Royal Danish Ballet), they were probably right.

In our experience, recovery from disordered eating is like this. The beginning is filled with awkward moments, fear of falling—and some actual falling. You might have heard "falls" referred to as setbacks, slipups, relapses, or simply lapses in behavior. We don't care what words you use. What is crucial is that, like Jenni's favorite Japanese proverb says, if you "fall down seven times," you "stand up eight." And the sooner you stand up, the better. It is easier to get back on track after one night of restricting (a lapse) than six weeks of bingeing and purging (a relapse).

At first, just standing back up is a triumph, but the next step is figuring out what knocked you down in the first place. Research has identified many predictors of eating disorder relapse. Some may seem obvious, like the persistence of body image disturbance, insufficient caloric intake, and excessive exercise after acute symptom remission.[9] Others are not directly related to food and weight—like work stress (such as being laid off), social stressors (such as breaking up with a close friend), and low overall psychosocial functioning—but nonetheless trigger disordered-eating behaviors.[10] The best way to identify your own individual triggers is to ask yourself immediately after a lapse, "Why did I feel compelled to return to a disordered-eating behavior just then?" When you've identified your triggers, start brainstorming ways to handle each of them in a healthy way.

Times of transition can be triggering to many people. For example, many students are fearful of gaining the dreaded "freshman fifteen" pounds during their first year on campus—even though such a gain is a myth.[11] Developing or returning to eating disorder symptoms is common in college. In one study, 49 percent of female students reported at least one symptom of disordered eating (such as strict dieting, bingeing, or purging) in the past year.[12] In a study of male undergraduates, 25 percent reported binge eating and 24 percent reported fasting in the past month.[13] Obviously, going to college is not the only transition that can be difficult. Others that can pose problems include getting divorced or even joyful times like getting married or having a baby. Keep in mind that just because certain times in life can be problematic does not mean that they have to be. Clinical psychologist Margo Maine told us, "I warn all my patients and their families about what I call 'the trouble with transitions.' Just as eating disorders initially develop at ages 13 to 15 and 17 to 19—during school transitions, physical changes in the body, and huge steps away from the family and into the world—we meet lots of transitions in adulthood and have little time or support to process these."[14] Surround yourself with social support to protect yourself during these times. And don't forget that you can be your own support, too, by practicing good self-care.

Watching out for yourself includes recognizing that slipping into destructive eating behaviors begins far before the actual bingeing, purging, or restricting. If you binge, for instance, the beginning of that setback might have actually happened days earlier when you let a friend take advantage of you. Stuffing your resentment—not reaching for the food—

might be considered the start of that binge. For this reason, one of the most effective relapse prevention strategies is to avoid getting to the place where you are on the verge of symptom use. To do this, you will need a recovery toolbox filled with tools that really work. If certain ideas and exercises in this book have been particularly helpful to you, consider listing them in your personalized relapse prevention plan in table 16 or in a notebook.

But I Keep Falling

Jenni's former dietitian, Reba Sloan, has explained, "Treating an eating disorder is like fighting a forest fire. We must put the entire fire out. If an 'ember' is still smoldering, there is a chance that the fire will be reignited."[15] If you keep falling into disordered-eating behaviors, maybe an ember of Ed is still burning in your life. Are you trying to keep your weight below a specific number? Is Ed still a coping mechanism? We all have a list of ways that we cope with life. To fully recover, Ed's name has to be taken off of that list completely. In the beginning, moving Ed's name to the bottom of the list is a great feat. But in the end, his name can't be scribbled in anywhere. Full freedom means that Ed is not an option. Period.

Sometimes, people have made promises to themselves about the circumstances under which they will truly commit to recovery. *I'll stop using eating-disordered behaviors when I graduate college. When I get married.* This is a trap. Samantha thought that she would give up her anorexia when she had a baby. But as long as she was too underweight to get her period, getting pregnant wasn't even a possibility.

If you keep lapsing into disordered-eating behaviors, you

Table 16.

Your Personalized Relapse Prevention Plan

Although different for everyone, common triggers for relapse include:

- events similar to those that first triggered the eating disorder (for example, others' comments about weight/shape, life transitions such as moving or graduating)
- unintentional weight gain (during pregnancy, for example) or loss (such as during a physical illness)
- events that increase focus on weight and shape (such as beach vacations or weddings)
- feeling like you have "failed" in another key life domain (such as a job or a relationship)
- negative mood (such as anxiety, depression, anger, frustration, or shame)

Which triggers are most likely to be relevant for me in the next 6 months?

_____

_____

What are the early warning signs that I am already starting to relapse?

- **Thoughts** (*such as "I should really lose 3 pounds before my date on Friday"*)

_____

_____

- **Feelings**

_____

_____

- **Behaviors** (*such as weighing myself frequently, eliminating specific food groups*)

_____

_____

What can I do to prevent a relapse from occurring?
- If you have gained or lost weight recently, write your feelings in your journal.
- If you are experiencing a negative mood, distract yourself with a fun task like knitting, watching a movie, or taking a yoga class, or express yourself by writing, drawing, or reaching out to a friend or family member face to face.
- If you have a stressful day, try meditation, deep breathing, or listening to music.
- Don't try to solve problems in unrelated life areas by changing your eating or weight. Such issues are part of life, no matter how thin or abstemious you are.
- If you feel a strong urge to use an eating-disordered behavior, experiment with setting a timer to delay for 10 minutes. Try one of the ideas listed in this section while you wait. By the time the buzzer rings, the urge may have passed.

Strategies that have worked for me in the past include:

_____

_____

What can I do to get back on track so a lapse doesn't become a full-blown relapse?
- Remind yourself that all is not lost! If you beat yourself up, you are promoting the same feelings of guilt and shame that put you at risk in the first place.
- Lapses are a great learning opportunity. Regroup and think about how you will handle the same situation differently next time.

Strategies that have worked for me in the past include:

_____

_____

might be trying to hold on to the "good" parts of almost anorexia while getting rid of the bad. But to get better, you cannot hold on to any part, which means saying good-bye to it all—even to the good. Remember from your "Friend" letter in chapter 6 that disordered eating serves a purpose in your life. Try rewriting that letter, which expressed gratitude to Ed, to also say good-bye. Letting go will be a grieving process, so feelings of sadness and even anger are common. But if you remain patient and stay the course with recovery, these feelings will usually pass.

When you first let go of almost anorexia, it might be helpful to remind yourself that you can always go back. Dr. Thomas often says to patients, "You have an impressive ability to restrict food, and no one can ever take that away from you. It's not like you're going to 'forget' how to be anorexic." Similarly, you can always go back to bingeing and purging if you make that choice. But our bet is that, once you experience the freedom of full recovery, you won't want to.

A Dream Big Enough to Beat Ed

You recover from an eating disorder in order to recover your life. This means that recovery will bring you face to face with your dreams. This is both exciting and scary. When you first start to feel better, you might wonder, like many people, *Who am I without my eating disorder?* This part of recovery is kind of like being placed in an empty room. The room is dull, not to mention uncomfortable, with no place to sit. But recovery is really about decorating the room. This is the fun part. You can fill up your room with anything at all—your favorite color, passions, relationships, and more.

Jenni's Journey

Earlier in this book, we compared embracing recovery to jumping out of an airplane and trusting that your parachute will open. This time, consider that disordered eating is a cliff. "Come over here. I can help you," the cliff called out to me. With such a promise and the beautiful view, I walked on over. And so I began living my life at the edge of the eating disorder cliff. As long as I could stay balanced on the edge, I felt in control—I was okay. But the cliff kept promising more and more, so I always got closer to the edge, eventually tumbling off to the rocky ground below—fully relapsing into disordered-eating behaviors. (The view doesn't look so great when you are plunging uncontrollably to the hard bottom.) Despite the falls, time and time again, I would pick myself up off the ground and walk right back to the alluring edge. Sometimes, I said that I wouldn't—*never again*—but I did. Maybe I was vulnerable to developing an eating-disorder cliff in the first place partly because I was born with personality traits like perfectionism and high anxiety. This was true, I realized, but I also learned that it couldn't be an excuse. Not anymore. (I was *not* born with an eating disorder but rather with these traits—an important difference.) To fully heal, I had to start taking purposeful steps away from the cliff. I stopped focusing on numbers like weight and calories. I promised to eat every day no matter what—a huge step. When I began utilizing my perfectionistic trait in a positive way, rather than using it to beat myself up, I made a gigantic leap. Harnessing the good in perfectionism means that I am driven. And I took yet another step when I became aware of my tendency toward anxiety and learned how not only to cope with it but also to refine it for good: I am dynamic! Today, I look around and see no cliff in sight. Sure, I might still stumble in life when difficulties arise, but I hit solid ground and stand back up again. I can't tumble off the cliff when it is nowhere near—and neither can you.

Discussing the more recent twenty-five-year follow-up interviews of women with anorexia and bulimia nervosa in the longitudinal study that we described earlier, Dr. Kamryn Eddy told us that one of the best indicators of recovery was redefining one's identity. She said, "Eating disorder recovery involves an attentional shift away from a self-worth based solely on weight, shape, eating, and their control and toward a sense of self that is founded in a broader collection of values and experiences. While the mechanisms of this progression from illness to wellness are difficult to describe, some women cite engagement in relationships—falling in love or having children, feeling connected with animals, and being valued at work—as experiences that impel this shift by giving their lives meaning."[16]

Jenni welcomes readers to post comments, questions, and words of inspiration on her Facebook and other social media pages. One particular post that caught her eye was from college student Amanda Olsen who said, "Finally found a dream big enough to beat Ed!" Battling Ed since middle school, Amanda had been through many ups and downs. In high school, her disordered eating even caused her to miss out on an opportunity to be a student ambassador in Japan—and she loved Japanese culture more than almost anything else. Years later when an opportunity arose yet again for Amanda to study abroad, Ed immediately said, "You can't do it." But then she asked herself, *Why not?* Amanda told us, "I realized then that all of my reasons for not being able to go were related to Ed, so for the first time, I genuinely wanted to get better for me. Since then, I've been working harder than ever before to achieve my dream."[17] Ultimately, Amanda was accepted to a university in Japan.

Do you have a dream big enough to beat Ed? You might have a dream for something you desire within the next five minutes *(to finish this chapter)*, five hours *(to eat your next meal)*, five days *(to buy clothes that fit your body now, not five pounds from now!)*, five months *(to go hiking in Costa Rica with your friends)*, or five years *(to be in a happy relationship with a partner other than Ed)*.

You might even consider making a list of all the dreams that Ed says are not possible for you. Then start doing those things and checking them off your list. One of Dr. Thomas's patients referred to this as her "recovery bucket list." Without Ed constantly telling her that she was fat, she could finally take a dance class, go on a date, and tell her recovery story at a local high school. Share your dream with us at www.jennischaefer.com.

People often ask us how they can share their recovery story in an effort to help others. There are all kinds of ways to share your story, but first ask yourself if you are ready. If talking with others about almost anorexia only triggers you to fall backward, then obviously it's not worth it. From experience, Jenni recommends that people wait to share their story until they have at least one year of solid recovery and also have experienced some success at avoiding relapse during difficult times. For some, their passion ultimately leads them to working professionally in the eating disorders field. If this is you, determine whether your desire is tied to an unhealthy need to stay connected with disordered eating *(If I can't have an Ed, I can at least talk with other people's Eds all day)* or if you genuinely want to help others. Guard against letting your "recovered" status define who you are as a person, even if it does end up being what you do as your job. Explaining his decision to specialize in eating disorders, physician Mark Warren, who is recovered himself, told us, "Given my visceral knowledge of the disorder, my optimism about recovery, my desire to have a more organized treatment world for those with whom I shared an experience, there was little else that held my attention like working in the eating disorder field." To help those considering following a similar path, he said, "This is not the right work if you feel triggered and unsafe. This is the right work for you if it gives you energy and makes you feel more whole."[18]

Never, Never, Never Give Up

Don't sell yourself short by getting halfway or even three quarters of the way better. Push past the various versions of "pseudorecovery"[19] to a complete one. It might be tempting, but try not to settle for even 99 percent better. Sure, we have heard people argue that they can survive in an almost-recovered phase, so why move further? And that might be true. But surviving and truly living are two different things.

You might be wondering how you will know when you are fully recovered. Hindsight often tells people when they are better, so try not to worry about exactly where you are along the way. Jenni, for instance, did not realize that she was fully recovered until friends and family started pointing it out. If your loved one is struggling, you can be a mirror like this—reflecting what you see, especially in terms of progress. When Jenni looked back at her life, she realized that she had been through many stressful periods without turning to eating-disordered behaviors (or even thinking about it). She discovered that she had formed genuine friendships and was living a joyful life. That's recovered. We have connected with countless men and women who have found this place of contentment and health. You can get there too.

Trade in jumping on the scale for jumping into life. This might surprise you, but a standard bathroom scale works, in large part, from one little spring, which snaps the dial back to zero when you step off. We have known people in recovery who have destroyed their scales, removed the spring, and then used it as a reminder to spring—not into body loathing, but into life. And that is exactly what recovering from disordered eating will help you to do. When Jenni first tried to get *Life Without Ed* published, literary agents and publishers were not interested. Okay, that's an understatement: she has a pile of more than fifty rejection letters at her house! Jenni did not quit despite this rejection, because she had already recovered from Ed, which was 100 times harder than facing this rejection. After you overcome almost anorexia—possibly one of the most difficult challenges you will ever face—something like a pile of rejection letters won't seem like a big deal. Your fresh perspective on life will move you in a different direction—one you never imagined possible. And with the tools from this book, you have the power to write a brand-new ending to your story.

appendix A

Summary of Diagnostic Criteria

The following appendix paraphrases the criteria listed in *DSM-5*, the *Diagnostic and Statistical Manual of Mental Disorders (5th edition)*, released by the American Psychiatric Association in May 2013.

DSM-5 Diagnostic Criteria for Anorexia Nervosa

A. Food restriction leading to a body weight that is substantially lower than normal or expected.

B. Very strong fear of weight gain, or repeated behavior that appears inconsistent with a stated desire to gain weight.

C. Inability to judge or perceive one's body accurately; overvaluation of shape or weight; or difficulty recognizing the health consequences of low weight.

Specify current subtype:

Restricting Type: No regular binge eating or purging (e.g., vomiting, laxatives, diuretics) for the past 3 months.

Binge-Eating/Purging Type: Regular binge eating or purging (e.g., vomiting, laxatives, diuretics) for the past 3 months.

Chapter 1: DSM-5 Subtypes of Other Specified Feeding and Eating Disorder (OSFED)

- **Atypical anorexia nervosa:** Meets criteria for anorexia nervosa, except that body weight is not substantially lower than normal or expected.

- **Subthreshold bulimia nervosa:** Meets criteria for bulimia nervosa, except that the binge eating and compensatory behaviors have taken place for fewer than three months, or occur less than once per week.

- **Subthreshold binge eating disorder:** Meets criteria for binge eating disorder, except that the binge eating has taken place for fewer than three months, or occurs less than once per week.

- **Purging disorder:** Regular purging (e.g., vomiting, laxatives, diuretics) at least once per week for at least three months, but in the absence of binge eating.

- **Night eating syndrome:** Repeated episodes of night eating, such as waking up in the middle of the night to eat, or consuming an excessive amount of calories after the evening meal. The night eating is remembered the next day, causes clinical impairment, and cannot be explained by social norms or another psychiatric disorder.

Unspecified feeding and eating disorder: An eating disorder of clinical severity that cannot be classified into any of the other specified feeding and eating disorder subtypes.

Chapter 3: DSM-5 Diagnostic Criteria for Bulimia Nervosa and Binge Eating Disorder

DSM-5 Bulimia Nervosa

A. Regular binge eating, defined as the consumption of a very large amount of food in a relatively short period of time, associated with perceived loss of control (i.e., the overeating feels unpreventable or unstoppable.

B. Regular compensatory behaviors that are intended to neutralize the impact of binge eating on shape and weight. These behaviors can include self-induced vomiting, use of laxatives, enemas, diuretics, stimulants, or diet pills, fasting, driven exercise, or any combination of these.

C. The binge eating and purging take place at least once per week for at least three months.

D. Overvaluation of shape and weight.

E. Criteria for anorexia nervosa are not met.

DSM-5 Binge Eating Disorder

A. Regular binge eating, defined as the consumption of a very large amount of food in a relatively short period of time, associated with perceived loss of control (i.e., the overeating feels unpreventable or unstoppable).

B. The binges are accompanied by at least three of these five features: eating very quickly, eating to uncomfortable fullness, eating when not hungry, eating alone due to shame, or feeling very upset after overeating.

C. The binge eating causes worry and concern.

D. The binges take place at least once per week for at least three months.

E. Criteria for anorexia nervosa or bulimia nervosa are not met.

appendix B

Self-Scoring

Chapter 1:
Scoring and Interpreting the EAT-26

Step 1: Attitudes. To calculate your total test score, assign yourself points for items 1 through 25 as follows:

- Always (3 points)
- Usually (2 points)
- Often (1 point)
- Sometimes (0 points)
- Rarely (0 points)
- Never (0 points)

Item 26 (no surprise, since it involves trying new, rich foods!) is scored in the opposite direction: Always (0 points), Usually (0 points), Often (0 points), Sometimes (1 point), Rarely (2 points), Never (3 points).

Now, you can add up your point value for each of the 26 items to obtain your total score.

Step 2: Body Weight. If you feel like you are in a good place (that is, Ed is not too excited about the idea of your making some calculations), you can determine your BMI with the following formula:

BMI = [Weight in pounds/(height in inches x height in inches)] x 703.

You can also determine your BMI online at the U.S. Department of Health and Human Services website (http://www.nhlbisupport.com/bmi/).

Step 3: Behaviors. Once you have calculated your total score, you can score each behavioral item individually. Give yourself 1 point if you have done any of the following in the past six months:

1. Had eating binges at least 2 to 3 times per month

2. Engaged in self-induced vomiting, laxative use, or diuretic use at least once a month

3. Exercised for 60 minutes to control weight every day

4. Lost 20 pounds

Under Age 18: Interpreting Your BMI

You can compare your BMI to child and adolescent norms created by the U.S. Centers for Disease Control. These norms provide percentiles based on the expected height and weight gain trajectories for sex and age, because the adult BMI ranges do not apply to growing children. You can find them at www.cdc.gov/healthyweight/assessing/bmi/childrens_bmi/about_childrens_bmi.html. If your BMI falls below the 5th percentile, then you are in the underweight range and may have anorexia nervosa. If your BMI falls below the 10th percentile and you need to actively restrict your intake to maintain this weight, you may have almost anorexia. As with adults, if your BMI falls in the normal (5th to 85th percentile), overweight (85th to 95th percentile), or obese (more than 95th percentile) range, and you do not meet criteria for bulimia or binge eating disorder, you may still have almost anorexia if you scored above the EAT-26 cutoffs in step 1 or 3, or if your preoccupation with eating or weight is impairing your life.

Chapter 8: Scoring and Interpreting the Compulsive Exercise Test

You can score the Compulsive Exercise Test by simply adding up all of the items to obtain a total score. The minimum possible score is 0 and the maximum possible score is 120. Although there is no specific cutoff, the higher your score, the more eating disordered your exercise behaviors are likely to be. For the two reverse-scored items (8 and 12), count a response of 0 as a response of 5, 1 as 4, 2 as 3, 3 as 2, 4 as 1, and 5 as 0. You can obtain specific subscale scores by adding up all of the items on that particular subscale, as follows. The higher your score on each subscale, the more problematic that area is for you:

- Avoidance and rule-driven behavior
  (items 9, 10, 11, 15, 16, 20, 22, 23)

- Weight-control exercise
  (items 2, 6, 8 [reverse-scored], 13, 18)

- Mood improvement
  (items 1, 4, 14, 17, 24)

- Lack of exercise enjoyment
  (items 5, 12 [reverse-scored], 21)

- Exercise rigidity (items 3, 7, 19)

appendix C

Seeking Professional Help

Here are some helpful resources for finding eating disorder specialists in your area:

Academy for Eating Disorders Referral List, www.aedweb.org (providers in the United States and around the world)

Beat Eating Disorders (Beat) HelpFinder Directory, www.b-eat.co.uk (providers in the United Kingdom and around the world)

Beat Helpline, 0845-634-1414, 0845-634-7650 for youth, United Kingdom

Binge Eating Disorder Association (BEDA), www.bedaonline.com (providers in the United States and around the world)

BEDA Helpline, 855-855-BEDA (2332), United States

Butterfly Foundation (resources in Australia), www.thebutterflyfoundation.org.au

Butterfly Foundation Support Line, 1-800-ED-HOPE (1-800-33-4673), Australia

Eating Disorder Referral and Information Center
www.edreferral.com
(providers in the United States and around the world)

FINDING*balance* **Gatherings** Find Christian eating
support groups at www.findingbalance.com.
FINDING*balance* is a nonprofit dedicated to providing
resources to people who struggle with all levels of
disordered eating.

**International Association of Eating Disorders Professionals
Foundation,** www.iaedp.com (providers in the United
States and around the world)

Multi-Service Eating Disorders Association, Inc. (MEDA),
www.medainc.org (providers in the United States)

**National Association of Anorexia Nervosa and Associated
Disorders Inc. (ANAD),** www.anad.org (providers in the
United States)

**National Eating Disorders Association (NEDA) Referral
List,** www.myneda.org (providers in the United States and
around the world)

NEDA Helpline, 1-800-931-2237, United States
(volunteers fluent in multiple languages)

National Eating Disorders Collaboration,
www.nedc.com.au (providers in Australia)

National Eating Disorder Information Centre,
www.nedic.ca (providers in Canada)

Supporting Treatment of Eating Disorders (F.E.A.S.T.)
www.feast-ed.org/
(support in the United States and around the world)

It's important to note that just because you see someone's name on a particular list does not mean that they are the best fit for you. Even a health insurance company's recommendation is not always appropriate. So, it will be necessary for you to interview professionals. Some questions to ask include these:

How long have you treated eating disorders? Do your best to locate a provider who specializes in eating disorders. Of course, having multiple years of experience is always a plus. However, don't disregard a less experienced clinician who has talent and enthusiasm for helping people with eating disorders. Sometimes, a new clinician who is very passionate can be quite effective. Be patient. It might take time to find the clinician who can best help you.

How many patients with eating disorders are currently in your practice? Some clinicians advertise that they treat eating disorders even if they see just one patient with an eating disorder every couple of years. Ideally, it would be great to work with someone who has a regular caseload of patients with eating disorders.

Do you use evidence-based treatment approaches? Although there is no one "right way" to treat eating disorders, certain approaches—such as family-based treatment for anorexia nervosa and cognitive-behavioral therapy for bulimia nervosa and EDNOS—have clear scientific support. Ask your prospective clinician whether he or she is knowledgeable about the latest advances in eating disorder treatment research.

Do you work with a team of other professionals? Eating disorders affect every facet of your life and body. A good clinician will collaborate with other professionals to make sure that all of your individual treatment needs are met.

. . .

If you live in an area where access to eating disorder specialists is limited or nonexistent, you will need to work toward educating your health care professionals. One way to do this is to give them a free, downloadable pamphlet created by the Academy for Eating Disorders titled *Eating Disorders: Critical Points for Early Recognition and Medical Risk Management in the Care of Individuals with Eating Disorders*, available at www.aedweb.org. You can also pass along this book or other helpful information.

Support and Therapy Group Resources

If you are looking to join an eating disorder support group, make sure you find a positive, pro-recovery one in which members are not tied to the identity of being sick but eagerly want to get better. The following resources can help you find a group in your area:

Beat Eating Disorders (Beat):
> The Beat Network includes a listing of groups in the United Kingdom at www.b-eat.co.uk.

Butterfly Foundation for Eating Disorders:
> Provides details for support groups located within Australia. See www.thebutterflyfoundation.org.au.

Eating Disorders Anonymous:

A Twelve Step program that promotes balance, not abstinence. Find free meetings in the United States as well as other countries at www.eatingdisordersanonymous.org.

National Association of Anorexia Nervosa and Associated Disorders Inc. (ANAD) Support Groups:

Locate free, peer-led groups in the United States at www.anad.org.

Therapy Groups:

Led by a licensed clinician and available for a fee, therapy groups might focus on a specific topic like body image or, alternatively, cover eating disorders in general. Certain treatment centers provide outpatient groups that are open to the public.

Resources to Help Pay for Treatment

Depending on your country's health care system, you may have difficulty affording treatment. Here are some tips for paying for care:

- Ask individual clinicians and treatment centers about scholarships and sliding-fee scales.

- If you have difficulty accessing health insurance benefits, download *Navigating and Understanding Health Insurance Issues* at www.myneda.org for free. This document is a part of a Toolkit for Parents developed by the National Eating Disorders Association (NEDA).

- Some organizations provide financial assistance for treatment, including:

- – F.R.E.E.D. Foundation, www.freedfoundation.org
- – Kirsten Haglund Foundation, www.kirstenhaglund
  .org
- – Manna Scholarship Fund, www.mannafund.org
- – Project HEAL, www.theprojectheal.org

- Research studies often offer free experimental treatments. Visit www.edreferral.com for a list of current opportunities.

• • •

If you think you need professional support, take steps to make an appointment. Even one Internet search or phone call can bring you closer to getting the help that you need. Be wary of programs, professionals, or groups that proclaim a quick fix for disordered eating. No therapist or organization can fix you, but they can certainly provide tools for you to help yourself.

notes

Introduction: A Touch of Anorexia

1. J. Arcelus, A. J. Mitchell, J. Wales, and S. Nielsen, "Mortality Rates in Patients with Anorexia Nervosa and Other Eating Disorders. A Meta-Analysis of 36 Studies," *Archives of General Psychiatry* 68 (2011): 724–31.

2. K. M. Flegal, M. D. Carroll, B. K. Kit, and C. L. Ogden, "Prevalence of Obesity and Trends in the Distribution of Body Mass Index among U.S. Adults, 1999–2010," *Journal of the American Medical Association* 307 (2012): 491–97.

3. American Psychiatric Association, *Diagnostic and Statistical Manual, 5th edition*, proposed diagnostic criteria for eating disorders. Retrieved May 31, 2012 from www.dsm5.org.

4. J. J. Thomas, L. R. Vartanian, and K. D. Brownell, "The Relationship between Eating Disorder Not Otherwise Specified (EDNOS) and Officially Recognized Eating Disorders: Meta-analysis and Implications for DSM," *Psychological Bulletin* 135 (2009): 407–33.

5. J. Schaefer and T. Rutledge, *Life Without Ed: How One Woman Declared Independence from Her Eating Disorder and How You Can Too* (New York: McGraw-Hill, 2003).

6. J. Schaefer, *Goodbye Ed, Hello Me: Recover from Your Eating Disorder and Fall in Love with Life* (New York: McGraw-Hill, 2009), 32.

7. A. Sterling, "No EDNOS in Sight: If Doctors Don't Fix the Problems with a Little-Known Disorder, Millions of Patients Will Continue to Suffer," *Shoe Leather Reported Stories*, June 2011, www.shoeleathermagazine.com /2011/sterling.shtml (accessed May 2, 2012).

Chapter 1: What Is Almost Anorexia?

1. D. A. Williamson, D. H. Gleaves, and T. M. Stewart, "Categorical versus Dimensional Models of Eating Disorders: An Examination of the Evidence," *International Journal of Eating Disorders* 37 (2005): 1–10.

2. C. G. Fairburn, *Cognitive Behavior Therapy and Eating Disorders* (New York: Guilford, 2008).

3. "Katie Couric: 'I Wrestled with Bulimia,'" *ABC News*, abcnews.go.com /blogs/entertainment/2012/09/katie-couric-i-wrestled-with-bulimia (accessed November 8, 2012).

4. J. Rodin, L. Silberstein, and R. Striegel-Moore, "Women and Weight: A Normative Discontent," *Nebraska Symposium and Motivation* 32 (1984): 267–307.

5. D. M. Garner, M. P. Olmstead, Y. Bohr, and P. E. Garfinkel, "The Eating Attitudes Test: Psychometric Features and Clinical Correlates," *Psychological Medicine* 12 (1982): 871–78.

6. B. Orbitello, R. Ciano, M. Corsaro, P. L. Rocco, C. Taboga, L. Tonutti, M. Armellini, and M. Balestrieri, "The EAT-26 as Screening Instrument for Clinical Nutrition Unit Attenders," *International Journal of Obesity* 30 (2006): 977–81; M. Siervo, V. Boschi, A. Papa, O. Bellini, and C. Falconi, "Application of the SCOFF, Eating Attitude Test 26 (EAT 26) and Eating Inventory (TFEQ) Questionnaires in Young Women Seeking Diet-Therapy," *Eating and Weight Disorders* 10 (2005): 76–82.

7. Associated Press, "Shaq Brushes Off Study," *ESPN NBA*, March 8, 2005, sports.espn.go.com/nba/news/story?id=2008024 (accessed May 30, 2012).

Chapter 2: Becoming Almost Anorexic

1. Jillian Lampert (Clinical Dietitian), email message with Jennifer J. Thomas, November 30, 2012.

2. Elijah Corbin (Eating Disorder Survivor), email message with Jenni Schaefer, August 12, 2012.

3. C. Arnold, *Next to Nothing: A Firsthand Account of One Teenager's Experience with an Eating Disorder* (Oxford: Oxford University Press, 2007), 55–56.

4. C. Rhodes, *Life Inside the "Thin" Cage: A Personal Look into the Hidden World of the Chronic Dieter* (Colorado Springs: WaterBrook Press, 2003), 110.

5. J. J. Thomas, L. R. Vartanian, and K. D. Brownell, "The Relationship between Eating Disorder Not Otherwise Specified (EDNOS) and Officially Recognized Eating Disorders: Meta-analysis and Implications for DSM." *Psychological Bulletin* 135 (3) (2009): 407–33.

6. A. E. Field, K. R. Sonneville, N. Micali, R. D. Crosby, S. A. Swanson, N. M. Laird, J. Treasure, R. Solmi, and N. J. Horton, "Prospective Association of Common Eating Disorders and Adverse Outcomes," *Pediatrics* 130 (2012): e289–95.

7. J. J. Thomas, "Newly Proposed DSM-5 Criteria Reduce the Need for 'Not Otherwise Specified' Diagnoses and Can Be Reliably Applied by Clinicians

in a Residential Eating Disorder Treatment Setting" (speech given at the International Conference on Eating Disorders, Austin, Texas, May 3–5, 2012).

8. M. Strober and M. Schneider, *Just a Little Too Thin: How to Pull Your Child Back from the Brink of an Eating Disorder* (Cambridge, MA: Da Capo Press, 2005).

9. S. Maguire, S. Touyz, L. Surgenor, R. D. Crosby, S. G. Engel, H. Lacey, S. Heywood-Everett, and D. L. Grange, "The Clinician Administered Staging Instrument for Anorexia Nervosa: Development and Psychometric Properties," *International Journal of Eating Disorders* 45 (2012): 390–99.

10. A. E. Andersen, W. A. Bowers, and T. Watson, "A Slimming Program for Eating Disorders Not Otherwise Specified: Reconceptualizing a Confusing, Residual Diagnostic Category," *Psychiatric Clinics of North America* 24 (2001): 271–80.

11. M. Hornbacher, *Wasted: A Memoir of Anorexia and Bulimia* (New York: HarperCollins, 1998), 180.

12. A. M. Bardone-Cone, "Examining the Match between Assessed Eating Disorder Recovery and Subjective Sense of Recovery," *European Eating Disorders Review* 20 (2011): 246–99.

13. A. Liu, *Gaining: The Truth about Life After Eating Disorders* (New York: Warner Books, 2007), 240.

14. A. E. Becker, R. A. Burwell, S. E. Gilman, D. B. Herzog, and P. Hamburg, "Eating Behaviours and Attitudes Following Prolonged Exposure to Television among Ethnic Fijian Adolescent Girls," *British Journal of Psychiatry* 180 (2002): 509–14.

15. A. E. Becker, J. J. Thomas, and K. M. Pike, "Should Non-Fat-Phobic Anorexia Nervosa Be Included in DSM-V?," *International Journal of Eating Disorders* 42 (2009): 620–35.

16. M. Strober, R. Freeman, C. Lampert, J. Diamond, and W. Kaye, "Controlled Family Study of Anorexia Nervosa and Bulimia Nervosa: Evidence of Shared Liability and Transmission of Partial Syndromes," *American Journal of Psychiatry* 157 (2000): 393–401.

17. K. L. Klump, J. L. Suisman, S. A. Burt, M. McGue, and W. G. Iacono, "Genetic and Environmental Influences on Disordered Eating: An Adoption Study," *Journal of Abnormal Psychology* 118 (2009): 797–805.

18. J. E. Dellava, L. M. Thornton, P. Lichtenstein, N. L. Pedersen, and C. M. Bulik, "Impact of Broadening Definitions of Anorexia Nervosa on Sample Characteristics," *Journal of Psychiatric Research* 45 (2011) 691–98.

19. C. M. Bulik, "Genetic Risk Factor for Eating Disorders," *Eating Disorders Review*, Fall 2007, http://www.eatingdisordersreview.com/nl/nl_edt_5_4_8. html (accessed October 18, 2012).

20. M. Chavez and T. R. Insel, "Eating Disorders: National Institute of Mental Health's Perspective," *American Psychologist* 62 (2007): 164.

21. L. C. Lyster-Mensh, "The Advantages of Brain Disorder Language from the Patient/Career Perspective" (paper presented at the International Conference on Eating Disorders, Austin, Texas, May 3–5, 2012).

22 L. Lilenfeld "Personality in Eating Disorders: Conceptual Understanding and Treatment Applications," (workshop at 2012 Renfrew Center Foundation Eating Disorders Conference for Professionals, November, 2012).

23. W. H. Kaye, "Neurobiology of Anorexia and Bulimia Nervosa," *Physiology & Behavior* 94 (2008): 121–35.

24. Walter Kaye (Psychiatrist), email message with Jenni Schaefer, October 26, 2012.

25. A. Zastrow, S. Kaiser, C. Stippich, S. Walther, W. Herzog, K. Tchanturia, A. Belger, M. Weisbrod, J. Treasure, and H. C. Friederich, "Neural Correlates of Impaired Cognitive-Behavioral Flexibility in Anorexia Nervosa," *American Journal of Psychiatry* 166 (2009): 608–16.

26. J. E. Steinglass, B. Finger, S. Berkowitz, H. B. Simpson, E. U. Weber, and B. T. Walsh, "Increased Capacity to Delay Reward in Anorexia Nervosa," *Journal of the International Neuropsychological Society* 18 (2012): 1–8.

27. S. E. Cassin and K. M. Von Ranson, "Personality and Eating Disorders: A Decade in Review," *Clinical Psychology Review* 25 (2005): 895–916.

28. S. Rosenfeld, "About me," http://everywomanhasaneatingdisorder.blogspot .com (accessed February 2, 2013).

29. D. Le Grange, S. A. Swanson, S. J. Crow, K. R. Merikangas, "Eating Disorder Not Otherwise Specified Presentation in the Population," *International Journal of Eating Disorders* 45 (2012): 711–18.

30. A. E. Field, K. R. Sonneville, N. Micali, R. D. Crosby, S. A. Swanson, N. M. Laird, J. Treasure, F. Solmi, and N. J. Horton, "Prospective Association of Common Eating Disorders and Adverse Outcomes," *Pediatrics* 130 (2012): e289–e95; and E. Stice, C. N. Marti, and P. Rohde, "Prevalence, Incidence, Impairment, and Course of the Proposed DSM-5 Eating Disorder Diagnoses in an 8-Year Prospective Community Study of Young Women," *Journal of Abnormal Psychology*, in press.

Chapter 3: Underweight, Overweight, and Everything in Between

1. A. B. de Gonzalez, P. Hartage, J. R. Cerhan, A. J. Flint, L. Hannan, R. J. Maclnnis, S. C. Moore, G. S. Tobias, H. Anton-Culver, L. B. Freeman, W. L. Beeson, S. L. Clipp, D. R. English, A. R. Folsom, D. M. Freedman, G. Giles, N. Hakansson, K. D. Henderson, J. Hoffman-Bolton, J. A. Hoppin, K. L. Koenig, I. Lee, M. S. Linet, Y. Park, G. Pocobelli, A. Schatzkin, H. D. Sesso, E. Weiderpass, B. J. Wilcox, A. Wolk, A. Zeleniuch-Jacquotte, W. C. Willett, and M. J. Thun, "Body-Mass Index and Mortality among 1.46 Million White Adults," *The New England Journal of Medicine* 363 (2010): 2211–19; and L. Dubois, K. O. Kyvik, M. Girard, F. Tatone-Tokuda, D. Perusse, J. Hjelmborg, A. Skytthe, F. Rasmussen, M. J. Wright, P. Lichtenstein, and N. G. Martin, "Genetic and Environmental Contributions to Weight, Height, and BMI from Birth to 19 Years of Age: An International Study of Over 12,000 Twin Pairs," *PLoS ONE* 7 (2012): e30153.

2. *Demi Lovato: Stay Strong* Documentary, MTV, March 6, 2012.

3. B. Timothy Walsh (Chair, *DSM-5* Eating Disorders Work Group), email message with Jennifer J. Thomas, October 23, 2012.

4. Adam Lamparello, Ten Mile Morning: My Journey Through Anorexia Nervosa (Lanham: Hamilton Books, 2012), 84–86.

5. J. J. Thomas, C. A. Roberto, and K. D. Brownell, "Eighty-Five Percent of What? Discrepancies in the Weight Cut-Off for Anorexia Nervosa Substantially Affect the Prevalence of Underweight," *Psychological Medicine* 39 (2009): 833–43.

6. B. Timothy Walsh (Chair, *DSM-5* Eating Disorders Work Group), email message with Jennifer J. Thomas, October 23, 2012.

7. D. Smeltzer, *Andrea's Voice: Silenced by Bulimia: Her Story and Her Mother's Journey Through Grief Toward Understanding* (Carlsbad, CA: Gurze Books, 2006).

8. Doris Smeltzer (mother of Andrea Smeltzer), email message with Jenni Schaefer, July 5, 2012.

9. S. J. Crow, C. B. Peterson, S. A. Swanson, N. C. Raymond, S. Specker, E. Eckert, and J. E. Mitchell, "Increased Mortality in Bulimia Nervosa and Other Eating Disorders," *American Journal of Psychiatry* 166 (2009): 1342–26.

10. D. A. Williamson, D. H. Gleaves, and T. M. Stewart, "Categorical versus Dimensional Models of Eating Disorders: An Examination of the Evidence," *International Journal of Eating Disorders* 37 (2005): 1–10.

11. D. Neumark-Sztainer, M. Wall, N. I. Larson, M. E. Eisenberg, and K. Loth, "Dieting and Disordered Eating Behaviors from Adolescence to Young Adulthood: Findings from a 10-Year Longitudinal Study," *Journal of the American Dietetic Association* 111 (2011): 1004–11.

12. J. E. Wildes, "Challenges to the Diagnostic Classification of Bulimia Nervosa: Partial-Syndrome Presentation and Comorbidity with Major Depression" (PhD dissertation, University of Oregon, 2004).

13. C. M. Bulik, M. D. Marcus, S. Zerwas, M. D. Levine, and M. La Via, "The Changing 'Weightscape' of Bulimia Nervosa," *American Journal of Psychiatry* 169 (2012): 1031–16.

14. Chevese Turner (Binge Eating Disorder Association President), email message with Jenni Schaefer, December 7, 2012.

15. C. M. Grilo, M. A. White, and R. M. Masheb, "Significance of Overvaluation of Shape and Weight in an Ethnically Diverse Sample of Obese Patients with Binge-Eating Disorder in Primary Care Settings," *Behaviour Research and Therapy* 50 (2012) 298–303.

16. E. Friedman, "Biggest Loser's Kai Hibbard Says Show Triggered Eating Disorder," *ABC News*, June 25, 2010, abcnews.go.com/Health/biggest-loser-contestant-kai-hibbard-eating-disorder/story?id=11012666#.UAIbl3BpZwk (accessed December 13, 2012).

17. G. Poretsky, "A Dose of Reality: My Exclusive Interview with Biggest Loser Finalist, Kai Hibbard (Part 2 of 3)," *Body Love Wellness*, June 16, 2010, www.bodylovewellness.com/2010/06/16/kai-hibbard-biggest-loser-finalist-part-2-of-3/ (accessed December 13, 2012).

18. N. Katz, "'Biggest Loser' Contestant Kai Hibbard Slams Reality Show, Gained Weight Back," CBS News, June 18, 2010, www.cbsnews.com/8301-504763_162-20008214-10391704.html (accessed December 13, 2012).

19. J. J. Thomas, K. T. Eddy, M. Gorman, S. Sogg, A. S. Hartmann, and A. E. Becker, "Newly Proposed DSM-5 Criteria Do Not Significantly Increase Eating Disorder Prevalence in Patients Seeking Treatment for Obesity" (paper presented at the Annual Meeting of the Eating Disorders Research Society, Porto, Portugal, September 20–22, 2012).

20. S. G. Engel, J. E. Mitchell, M. de Zwaan, and K. J. Steffen, "Eating Disorders and Eating Problems Pre- and Postbariatric Surgery," in *Psychosocial Assessment and Treatment of Bariatric Surgery Patients*, ed. James E. Mitchell and Martina de Zwaan (New York: Routledge, 2012), 61–85.

21. D. Neumark-Sztainer, M. Wall, M. Story, and A. R. Standish, "Dieting and Unhealthy Weight Control Behaviors during Adolescence: Associations

with 10-Year Changes in Body Mass Index," *Journal of Adolescent Health* 50 (2012): 80–86.

22. J. J. Thompson-McCormick, J. J. Thomas, A. Bainivualiku, A. N. Khan, and A. E. Becker, "Breakfast Skipping as a Risk Correlate for Overweight and Obesity in School-Going Ethnic Fijian Adolescent Girls," *Asia Pacific Journal of Clinical Nutrition* 19 (2010): 372–82.

23. K. H. Pietilainen, S. E. Saarni, J. Kaprio, and A. Rissanen, "Does Dieting Make You Fat? A Twin Study," *International Journal of Obesity* 36 (2012): 456–64.

24. P. Sumithran, L. A. Prendergast, E. Delbridge, K. Purcell, A. Shulkes, A. Kriketos, and J. Proietto, "Long-Term Persistence of Hormonal Adaptations to Weight Loss," *New England Journal of Medicine* 365 (2011): 1597–604.

25. L. Bacon, *Health at Every Size: The Surprising Truth about Your Weight* (Dallas: BenBella Books, 2010), 307.

26. Z. Edwards, "Are You Guilty of Gorging on Diet Show? Supersize vs Superskinny Said to Be a 'Trigger' for Eating Disorder Sufferers," *Daily Mail*, February 15, 2012, www.dailymail.co.uk/tvshowbiz/article-2098744/Supersize-vs-Superskinny-said-trigger-eating-disorder-sufferers.html (accessed November 5, 2012).

27. D. L. McGee, "Body Mass Index and Mortality: A Meta-analysis Based on Person-level Data from Twenty-Six Observational Studies," *Annals of Epidemiology* 15 (2005): 87–97.

28. K. M. Flegal, B. I. Graubard, D. F. Williamson, and M. H. Gail, "Excess Deaths Associated with Underweight, Overweight, and Obesity," *The Journal of the American Medical Association* 293 (2005): 1861–17.

29. R. Chastain, *Fat: The Owner's Manual* (Austin, TX: Sized for Success Multimedia, LLC, 2012).

30. R. Chastain (Self-Acceptance Blogger), email message with Jenni Schaefer, March 27, 2012.

31. M. G. Cooper, K. Deepak, E. Grocutt, and E. Baily, "The Experience of 'Feeling Fat' in Women with Anorexia Nervosa, Dieting and Non-dieting Women: An Exploratory Study," *European Eating Disorders Review* 15 (2007): 366–72.

32. Fairburn, *Cognitive Behavior Therapy and Eating Disorders*, 114.

33. Ibid., 115.

Chapter 4: Calories, Cleansing, and Colonics, Oh My! Your Relationship with Food

1. A. G. Walton, "The Feeding Tube Diet and Our Limitless Weight-
Loss Idiocy," *Forbes*, April 17, 2012, www.forbes.com/sites/alicegwalton
/2012/04/17/the-feeding-tube-diet-and-our-limitless-weight-loss-idiocy
(accessed October 7, 2012).

2. N. Habgood, *The No Diet, Diet!* (Bloomington, IN: AuthorHouse, 2007).

3. J. J. S. Chafen, S. J. Newberry, M. A. Riedl, D. M. Bravata, M. Maglione,
M. J. Suttorp, V. Sundaram, N. M Paige, A. Towfigh, B. J. Hulley, and
P. G. Shekelle, "Diagnosing and Managing Common Food Allergies: A
Systematic Review," *Journal of the American Medical Association* 303 (2010):
1848–56.

4. A. Rubio-Tapia, J. F. Ludvigsson, T. L. Brantner, J. A. Murray, and J. E.
Everhart, "The Prevalence of Celiac Disease in the United States," *American
Journal of Gastroenterology* 107 (2012): 1538–44.

5. J. A. Boyce, A. Assa'ad, A. W. Burks, S. M. Jones, H. A. Sampson, R.
A. Wood, M. Plaut, S. F. Cooper, and M. J. Fenton, "Guidelines for
the Diagnosis and Management of Food Allergies in the United States:
Summary of the NIAD-Sponsored Expert Panel Report," *Journal of the
American Dietetic Association* 111 (2011): 17–27.

6. Jaimie Winkler (Dietitian), email message with Jennifer J. Thomas, October
15, 2012.

7. A. N. Gearhardt, S. Yokum, P. T. Orr, E. Stice, W. R. Corbin, and K.
D. Brownell, "Neural Correlates of Food Addiction," *Archives of General
Psychiatry* 68 (2011) 808–16.

8. A. N. Gearhardt, C. M. Grilo, R. J. DiLeone, K. D. Brownell, and M. N.
Potenza, "Can Food Be Addictive? Public Health and Policy Implications,"
Addiction 106 (2011): 1208–12.

9. A. M. Bardone-Cone, E. E. Fitzsimmons-Craft, M. B. Harney, C. R.
Maldonado, M. A. Lawson, R. Smith, and D. P. Robinson, "The Inter-
relationships between Vegetarianism and Eating Disorders among Females,"
Journal of the Academy of Nutrition and Dietetics 112 (2012): 1247–52.

10. F. Patenaude, *Raw Food Controversies: How to Avoid Common Mistakes that
May Sabotage Your Health* (Montreal: CreateSpace, 2011), 174.

11. Ibid., 67.

12. C. Koebnick, A. L. Garcia, P. C. Dagnelie, C. Strassner, J. Lindemans,
N. Katz, C. Leitzmann, and I. Hoffman, "Long-Term Consumption of a
Raw Food Diet Is Associated with Favorable Serum LDL Cholesterol and

Triglycerides but Also with Elevated Plasma Homocysteine and Low Serum HDL Cholesterol in Humans," *Journal of Nutrition* 135 (2005): 2372–28.

13. C. Boone O'Neill, *Starving for Attention* (New York: Continuum, 1982), xi.

14. C. R. Rabin, "Rabbis Sound Alarm over Eating Disorders," *New York Times*, April 12, 2011, www.nytimes.com/2011/04/12/health/12orthodox.html (accessed October 9, 2012).

15. J. A. Mattison, G. S. Roth, M. Beasley, E. M. Tilmont, A. M. Handy, R. L. Herbert, D. L. Longo, D. B. Allison, J. E. Young, M. Bryant, D. Barnard, W. F. Ward, W. Qi, D. K. Ingram, and R. de Cabo, "Impact of Caloric Restriction on Health and Survival in Rhesus Monkeys from the NIA Study," *Nature* 489 (2012): 318–22.

16. K. M. Vitousek, J. A. Gray, and K. M, Grubbs, "Caloric Restriction for Longevity I; Paradigm, Protocols and Physiological Findings in Animal Research," *European Eating Disorders Review* 12 (2004): 285.

17. L.A. Neighbors and J. Sobal, "Weight and Weddings: Women's Weight Ideals and Weight Management Behaviors for Their Wedding Day," *Appetite* 50 (2008): 550–54.

18. S. Bratman, *Health Food Junkies: Overcoming the Obsession with Healthful Eating* (New York: Broadway Books, 2000), 65.

19. J. Mathieu, "What Is Preguorania?" *Journal of the American Dietetic Association* 109 (2009): 976–79.

20. C. M. Bulik, *The Woman in the Mirror: How to Stop Confusing What You Look Like with Who You Are* (New York: Walker, 2011).

21. E. Susser, H. W. Hoek, and A. Brown, "Neurodevelopmental Disorders after Prenatal Famine: The Story of the Dutch Famine Study," *American Journal of Epidemiology* 147 (1998): 213-6.

22. S. M. Giles, H. Champion, E. L. Sutfin, T. P. McCoy, and K, Wagoner, "Calorie Restriction on Drinking Days: An Examination of Drinking Consequences among College Students," *Journal of American College Health* 57 (2009) 603–09.

23. *Heathers*, directed by M. Lehman, 1988, CA, USA: Anchor Bay Entertainment, 2001, DVD.

24. W. H. Kaye, T. E. Weltzin, G. Hsu, C. W. McConaha, and B. Bolton, "Amount of Calories Retained after Binge Eating and Vomiting," *American Journal of Psychiatry* 150 (1993): 969–71; and G. W. Bo-Linn, C. A. Santa Ana, S. G. Morawski, and J. S. Fordtran, "Purging and Calorie Absorption in Bulimic Patients and Normal Weight Women," *Annals of Internal Medicine* 99 (1983): 14–17.

25. P. K. Keel, T. F. Heatherton, D. J. Dorer, T. E. Joiner, and A. K. Zalta, "Point Prevalence of Bulimia Nervosa in 1982, 1992, and 2002," *Psychological Medicine* 36 (2006): 119–27; and L. Currin, U. Schmidt, J. Treasure, and H. Jick, "Time Trends in Eating Disorder Incidence," *British Journal of Psychiatry* 186 (2005): 132–25.

26. K. Matthews, "Master Cleanse Garners Praise, Criticism," *The Washington Post*, May 2, 2007, www.washingtonpost.com/wp-dyn/content/article /2007/05/02/AR2007050201401.html (accessed October 10, 2012).

27. A. M. Johnstone, "Fasting—the Ultimate Diet?" *Obesity Reviews* 8 (2007): 211–22.

28. J. J. Thomas, R. D. Crosby, S. A. Wonderlich, R. H. Striegel-Moore, and A. E. Becker, "A Latent Profile Analysis of the Typology of Bulimic Symptoms in an Indigenous Pacific Population: Evidence of Cross-Cultural Variation in Phenomenology," *Psychological Medicine* 41 (2011): 195–206.

29. R. Mishori, A. Otubu, and A. A. Jones, "The Dangers of Colon Cleansing," *The Journal of Family Practice* 60 (2011): 454–57.

30. A. E. Goebel-Fabbri, J. Fikkan, D. L. Franko, K. Pearson, B. J. Anderson, and K. Weinger, "Insulin Restriction and Associated Morbidity and Mortality in Women with Type I Diabetes," *Diabetes Care* 31 (2008): 415–19.

Chapter 5: Optical Illusions: Your Relationship with Your Body

1. M. Nichter, *Fat Talk: What Girls and Their Parents Say about Dieting* (USA: Harvard University Press, 2001).

2. *Mean Girls*, directed by M. Waters, LA, CA: Paramont Studios, 2004, DVD.

3. S. Hayes and S. Tantleff-Dunn, "Am I Too Fat to Be a Princess? Examining the Effects of Popular Children's Media on Young Girls' Body Image," *British Journal of Developmental Psychology* 28 (2010): 413–26.

4. D. School and L. S. Lowry, "Hispanic/Latino Body Images," in *Body Image, Second Edition: A Handbook of Science, Practice, and Prevention*, eds. T. F. Cash and L. Smolak (New York: Guilford, 2011), 237–43.

5. A. M. Darcy, A. C. Doyle, J. Lock, R. Peebles, P. Doyle, and D. Le Grange, "The Eating Disorders Examination in Adolescent Males with Anorexia Nervosa: How Does It Compare to Adolescent Females?" *International Journal of Eating Disorders* 45 (2012): 110–14.

6. S. B. Murray, E. Rieger, S. W. Touyz, and Y. D. Garcia, "Muscle Dysmorphia and the DSM-V Conundrum: Where Does It Belong? A Review Paper," *International Journal of Eating Disorders* 43 (2010): 483–91.

7. A. S. Hartmann, J. L. Greenberg, and S. Wilhelm, "The Relationship between Anorexia Nervosa and Body Dysmorphic Disorder" *Clinical Psychology Review*, in press.

8. H. Pope, K. A. Phillips, and R. Olivardia, *The Adonis Complex: The Secret Crisis of Male Body Obsession* (New York: Free Press, 2000), 5.

9. L. A. Peplau, D. A. Frederick, C. Yee, N. Maisel, J. Lever, and N. Ghavami, "Body Image Satisfaction in Heterosexual, Gay, and Lesbian Adults," *Archives of Sexual Behavior* 38 (2009): 713–25.

10. Brad Kennington, LMFT, email message with Jenni Schaefer, October 18, 2012.

11. D. Keeps, "Get a Peek Inside Cindy Crawford's Home," *Redbook*, www.redbookmag.com/fun-contests/celebrity/celeb-pics/cindy-crawford -interview (accessed October 27, 2012).

12. Roy A. Cui (Digital Artist), email message with Jenni Schaefer, October 19, 2012.

13. Sarah Ziff (Fashion Model), email message with Jenni Schaefer, October 29, 2012.

14. L. Hardy, "A Big Fat (and Very Dangerous) Lie: A Former Cosmo Editor Lifts the Lid on Airbrushing Skinny Models to Look Healthy," *Daily Mail*, May 20, 2010, www.dailymail.co.uk/femail/article-1279766/Former -Cosmo-editor-LEAH-HARDY-airbrushing-skinny-models-look-healthy -big-fat-dangerous-lie.html (accessed October 27, 2012).

15. K. C. Taber, "With Model's Death, Eating Disorders Are Again in Spotlight," *New York Times*, November 20, 2006, www.nytimes. com/2006/11/20/world/americas/20iht-models.3604439.html (accessed November 5, 2012); W. Grimes, "Isabelle Caro, Anorexic Model, Dies at 28," *New York Times*, December 31, 2010, www.nytimes.com/2010/12/31 /world/europe/31caro.html (accessed November 5, 2012); and A. Levy, "Anorexia Tragedy of Teenage Cover Girl: Parents Tell of Their Grief over 19-Year-Old Who 'Didn't Realise How Beautiful She Was'," *Daily Mail*, April 20, 2012, www.dailymail.co.uk/news/article-2137423/Bethaney -Wallace-Anorexic-cover-girl-model-19-dies-sleep-weight-drops-6-stone .html (accessed November 5, 2012).

16. Hardy, "A Big Fat (and Very Dangerous) Lie: A Former Cosmo Editor Lifts the Lid on Airbrushing Skinny Models to Look Healthy."

17. A. Slater, M. Tiggemann, B. Firth, and K. Hawkins, "Reality Check: An Experimental Investigation of the Addition of Warning Labels to Fashion Magazine Images on Women's Mood and Body Dissatisfaction," *Journal of Social and Clinical Psychology* 31 (2012): 105–22.

18. G. Smith, "Backlash after Australian Newspaper Describes Olympic Triple-Gold Medallist as Fat and Questions Her Fitness," *Mail Online*, www.dailymail.co.uk/news/article-2179394/Backlash-Australian-newspaper -describes-Olympic-triple-gold-medallist-fat-questions-fitness.html.

19. J. Springer, "I'm Not Fat, Says Ballerina Faulted for 'Too Many Sugar- plums'," *Today News*, December 13, 2010, www.today.msnbc.msn.com /id/40639920/ns/today-today_news/t/im-not-fat-says-ballerina-faulted -too-many-sugarplums/#.UI2YLKkZfww (accessed December 13, 2012).

20. "Adele's Health Crisis and Comeback," *People*, February 8, 2012, www .peoplestylewatch.com/people/stylewatch/package/article/0,,20552371 _20568143,00.html (accessed October 28, 2012).

21. J. Haines, D. Neumark-Sztainer, M. E. Eisenberg, and P. J. Hannan, "Weight Teasing and Disordered Eating Behaviors in Adolescents: Longitudinal Findings from Project EAT (Eating among Teens)," *Pediatrics* 117 (2006): e209–e15.

22. The Center for Eating Disorders at Sheppard Pratt, "Public Survey Conducted by the Center for Eating Disorders at Sheppard Pratt Finds Facebook Use Impacts the Way Many People Feel about Their Bodies," *PR Newswire*, press release March 28, 2012, www.prnewswire.com/news -releases/public-survey-conducted-by-the-center-for-eating-disorders -at-sheppard-pratt-reveals-that-facebook-drains-body-image-and-self -esteem-144601505.html (accessed August 3, 2012).

23. J. Geller, C. Johnston, and K. Madsen, "The Role of Shape and Weight in Self-Concept: The Shape and Weight Based Self-Esteem Inventory," *Cognitive Therapy and Research* 21 (1997): 5–24.

24. Fairburn, *Cognitive Behavior Therapy and Eating Disorders*, 96.

25. J. Geller, C. Johnston, K. Madsen, E. M. Goldner, R. A. Remick, and C. L. Birmingham, "Shape- and Weight-Based Self-Esteem and the Eating Disorders," *International Journal of Eating Disorders* 24 (1998): 285–98; and S. M Wilksch and T. D. Wade, "Risk Factors for Clinically Significant Importance of Shape and Weight in Adolescent Girls," *Journal of Abnormal Psychology* 119 (2010): 206–15.

26. Fairburn, Cognitive Behavior Therapy and Eating Disorders, 99.

27. A. Jansen, C. Nederkoom, and S. Mulkens, "Selective Visual Attention for Ugly and Beautiful Body Parts in Eating Disorders," *Behaviour Research and Therapy* 43 (2005) 183–96.

28. D. Cabrera and E. T. Wierenga, *Mom in the Mirror: Body Image, Beauty, and Life after Pregnancy* (USA: Rowman & Littlefield, 2013).

29. Emily Wierenga (Artist), email message with Jenni Schaefer, November 26, 2012.

30. R. Shafran, C. G. Fairburn, P. Robsinson, and B. Lask, "Body Checking and Its Avoidance in Eating Disorders," *International Journal of Eating Disorders* 35 (2004): 93–101.

31. D. L. Reas, B. L. Whisenhunt, R. Netemeyer, and D. A. Williamson, "Development of the Body Checking Questionnaire: A Self-Report Measure of Body Checking Behaviors," *International Journal of Eating Disorders* 31 (2002): 324–33.

32. T. Hildebrandt, D. C. Walker, L. Alfano, S. Delinsky, and K. Bannon, "Development and Validation of a Male Specific Body Checking Questionnaire," *International Journal of Eating Disorders* 43 (2010): 77–87.

33. J. J. Thomas, T. J. Weigel, B. Lawton, P. G. Levendusky, and A. E. Becker, "The Cognitive-Behavioral Treatment of Body Image Disturbance in a Congenitally Blind Patient with Anorexia Nervosa," *American Journal of Psychiatry*, in press.

34. Becker, Thomas, and Pike, "Should Non-Fat-Phobic Anorexia Nervosa Be Included in DSM-V?"

Chapter 6: Resisting the Allure of Almost Anorexia

1. J. J. Brumberg, *Fasting Girls: The History of Anorexia Nervosa* (USA: Vintage, 2000).

2. S. Hogan, "Drive-Thru Guru: Wiley Brooks Says He Has Discovered the Secrets to Immortality, and One of Them Is on the Dollar Menu," *The Times*, www.timespublications.com/jun10-feature1.asp (accessed October 14, 2012).

3. V. Bauman, "Wannarexic Girls Yearn for Eating Disorders," *USA Today*, August 4, 2007, www.usatoday.com/news/health/2007-08-04-wannarexic _N.htm (accessed October 10, 2012).

4. C. Gale, J. Holliday, N. Troop, L. Serpell, and J. Treasure, "Pros and Cons of Change in Individuals with Eating Disorders: A Broader Perspective," *International Journal of Eating Disorders* 39 (2006): 394–403.

5. C. Gregoire, "The Hunger Blogs: A Secret World of Teenage Thinspiration," Huffington Post, February 9, 2012 www.huffingtonpost.com/2012/02/08/thinspiration-blogs_n_1264459.html (accessed October 10, 2012).

6. C. H. Andersen, "Is 'Fitspiration' Really Any Better Than 'Thinspiration'?" The Great Fitness Experiment, February 26, 2012, www.thegreatfitnessexperiment.com/2012/02/is-fitspiration-really-any-better-than-thinspiration.html (accessed October 14, 2012).

7. A. M. Bardone-Cone and K. M. Cass, "What Does Viewing a Pro-Anorexia Website Do? An Experimental Examination of Website Exposure and Moderating Effects," *International Journal of Eating Disorders* 40 (2007): 537–48.

8. K. Homan, E. McHugh, D. Wells, C. Watson, and C. King, "The Effect of Viewing Ultra-Fit Images on College Women's Body Dissatisfaction," *Body Image* 9 (2012) 9: 50–56.

9. M. B. Schwartz, J. J. Thomas, K. M. Bohan, and L. R. Vartanian, "Intended and Unintended Effects of an Eating Disorder Educational Program: The Impact of Presenter Identity," *International Journal of Eating Disorders* 40 (2007): 187–92.

10. J. J Thomas, A. M. Judge, K. D. Brownell, and L. R. Vartanian, "Evaluating the Effects of Eating Disorder Memoirs on Readers' Eating Attitudes and Behaviors," *International Journal of Eating Disorders* 39 (2006): 418–25.

11. E. Lamont, L. R. Vartanian, and J. J. Thomas, "Readers of Eating Disorder Memoirs Recall More Positive Than Negative Aspects of Eating Disorders," unpublished manuscript.

12. S. K. O'Hara and K. G. Smith, "Presentation of Eating Disorders in the News Media: What Are the Implications for Patient Diagnosis and Treatment?," *Patient Education and Counseling* 68 (2007): 48.

13. V. Mainz, M. Schulte-Ruther, G. R. Fink, B. Herpertz-Dahlmann, and K. Konrad, "Structural Brain Abnormalities in Adolescent Anorexia Nervosa Before and After Weight Recovery and Associated Hormonal Changes," *Psychosomatic Medicine* 74 (2012): 574–82.

14. Y. Y. Choi, N. A. Shamosh, S. H. Cho, C. G. DeYoung, M. J. Lee, J. M. Lee , S. I. Kim, Z. H. Cho, K. Kim, J. R. Gray, and K. H. Lee, "Multiple Bases of Human Intelligence Revealed by Cortical Thickness and Neural Activation," *Journal of Neuroscience* 28 (2008): 10323–29.

15. R. Peebles, K. K. Hardy, J. L. Wilson, and J. D. Lock, "Are Diagnostic Criteria for Eating Disorders Markers of Medical Severity?" *Pediatrics* 125 (2010): e1193–201.

16. J. I. Hudson, J. K. Lalonde, C. E. Coit, M. T. Tsuang, S. L. McElroy, S. J. Crow, C. M. Bulik, M. S. Hudson, J. A. Yanovski, N. R. Rosenthal, and H. G. Pope Jr., "Longitudinal Study of the Diagnosis of Components of the Metabolic Syndrome in Individuals with Binge-Eating Disorder," *American Journal of Clinical Nutrition* 91 (2009): 1568–73.

17. Ovidio Bermudez (Pediatrician), email message with Jenni Schaefer, October 19, 2012.

18. K. Bohn and C. G. Fairburn, "The Clinical Impairment Assessment Questionnaire (CIA 3.0)," in *Cognitive Behavior Therapy and Eating Disorders*, ed. C. G. Fairburn (New York: Guilford Press, 2008).

19. D. M. Garner, "Psychoeducational Principles in Treatment," in *Handbook of Treatment for Eating Disorders*, eds. D. M. Garner and P. E. Garfinkle (New York: Guilford, 1997), 145–77.

20. C. M. Nevins, K. T. Eddy, and J. J. Thomas, "Diagnostic Crossover," in *Anorexia: Symptoms, Treatment and Neurobiology*, ed. N. C. Marsteller (New York: Nova, 2012), 1–22.

21. *Someday Melissa*, directed by J. Cobelli, 2011, USA: Good For You Productions, 2011, DVD.

22. L. Forcano, E. Alvarez, J. J. Santamaria, S. Jimenez-Murcia, R. Granero, F. Penelo, P. Alonso, I. Sanchez, J. M. Menchon, E. Ullman, C. M. Bulik, and F. Fernandez-Aranda, "Suicide Attempts in Anorexia Nervosa Subtypes," *Comprehensive Psychiatry* 52 (2011): 352–58.

23. S. S. Delinsky, J. J. Thomas, S. A. St. Germain, T. J. Weigel, P. G. Levendusky, and A. E. Becker, "Motivation to Change among Residential Treatment Patients with an Eating Disorder: Assessment of Multi-dimensionality of Motivation and Its Relation to Treatment Outcome," *International Journal of Eating Disorders* 44 (2011) 340–48.

24. L. Serpell, J. Treasure, J. Teasdale, and V. Sullivan, "Anorexia Nervosa: Friend or Foe?" *International Journal of Eating Disorders* 25 (1999): 177–86.

Chapter 7: Do the Next Right Thing: Normal Eating

1. Fairburn, *Cognitive Behavior Therapy and Eating Disorders*.

2. D. Neumark-Sztainer, M. E. Eisenberg, J. A. Fulkerson, M. Story, and N. I. Larson, "Family Meals and Disordered Eating in Adolescents: Longitudinal Findings from Project EAT," *Archives Pediatric Adolescent Medicine* 162 (2008): 17–22.

3. J. Lock, D. Le Grange, W. S. Agras, and C. Dare, *Treatment Manual for Anorexia Nervosa: A Family-Based Approach* (New York: Guilford, 2001);

and C. M. Bulik, D. H. Baucom, J. S. Kirby, and E. Pisetsky, "Uniting Couples (in the Treatment of) Anorexia Nervosa (UCAN)," *International Journal of Eating Disorders* 44 (2011): 19–28.

4. H. Brown, *Brave Girl Eating: A Family's Struggle with Anorexia* (New York: HarperCollins, 2010), 192.

5. L. Craighead, *The Appetite Awareness Workbook: How to Listen to Your Body and Overcome Bingeing, Overeating, and Obsession with Food* (Oakland: New Harbinger Publications, 2006), 54.

6. P. S. Mehler, A. B. Winkelman, D. M. Andersen, and J. L. Gaudiani, "Nutritional Rehabilitation: Practical Guidelines for Refeeding the Anorectic Patient," *Journal of Nutrition and Metabolism 2010* (2010), doi:10.1155/2010/625782.

7. E. Tribole, "Intuitive Eating in the Treatment of Eating Disorders: The Journal of Attunement," *Perspectives: A Professional Journal of the Renfrew Treatment Foundation* (Winter 2010) 11–4.

8. L. Benini, T. Todesco, R. Dalle Grave, F. Deiorio, L. Salandini, and I. Vantini, "Gastric Emptying in Patients with Restricting and Binge/Purging Subtypes of Anorexia Nervosa," *American Journal of Gastroenterology* 99 (2004): 1448–54.

9. A. Santonicola, M. Siniscalchi, P. Capone, S. Gallotta, C. Ciacci, and P. Iovino, "Prevalence of Functional Dyspepsia and Its Subgroups in Patients with Eating Disorders," *World Journal of Gastroenterology* 32 (2012): 4379–85.

10. C. Zunker, C. B. Peterson, R. D. Crosby, L. Cao, S. G. Engel, J. E. Mitchell, and S. A. Wonderlich, "Ecological Momentary Assessment of Bulimia Nervosa: Does Dietary Restriction Predict Binge Eating?," *Behaviour Research and Therapy* 49 (2011): 714–47.

11. D. Urbszat, C. P Herman, and J. Polivy, "Eat, Drink, and Be Merry, for Tomorrow We Diet: Effects of Anticipated Deprivation on Food Intake in Restrained and Unrestrained Eaters," *Journal of Abnormal Psychology* 2 (2002): 396–401.

12. K. C. Berg, R. D. Crosby, L. Cao, C. B. Peterson, S. G. Engel, J. E. Mitchell, and S. A. Wonderlich, "Facets of Negative Affect Prior to and Following Binge-Only, Purge-Only, and Binge/Purge Events in Women With Bulimia Nervosa," *Journal of Abnormal Psychology*, in press.

13. T. L. Tylka, "Development and Psychometric Evaluation of a Measure of Intuitive Eating," *Journal of Counseling Psychology* 53 (2006) 226–40.

14. E. Tribole and E. Resch, *Intuitive Eating: A Revolutionary Program That Works* (New York: St. Martin's Griffin, 2012), 14.

15. J. S. Coelho, J. C. Carter, T. McFarlane, and J. Polivy, "'Just Looking at Food Makes Me Gain Weight': Experimental Induction of Thought-Shape Fusion in Eating-Disordered and Non-Eating-Disordered Women," *Behaviour Research and Therapy* 46 (2008): 219–28.

16. Ed Tyson (Physician), email message with Jenni Schaefer, October 20, 2012.

17. D. M. Hill, L. W. Craighead, and D. L. Safer, "Appetite-Focused Dialectical Behavior Therapy for the Treatment of Binge Eating with Purging: A Preliminary Trial," *International Journal of Eating Disorders* 44 (2011): 249–61; and K. N. Boutelle, N. L. Zucker, C. B. Peterson, S. A. Rydell, G. Cafri, and L. Harnack, "Two Novel Treatments to Reduce Overeating in Overweight Children: A Randomized Controlled Trial," *Journal of Consulting and Clinical Psychology* 79 (2011): 759–71.

18. S. Hart, S. Abraham, R. C. Franklin, and J. Russell, "The Reasons Why Eating Disorder Patients Drink," *European Eating Disorders Review* 19 (2011): 121–28.

19. E. N. Harrop and G. A. Marlatt "The Comorbidity of Substance Use Disorders and Eating Disorders in Women: Prevalence, Etiology, and Treatment," *Addictive Behaviors* 35(2010): 392–98.

20. G. Waller, H. Cordery, E. Corstorphine, H. Hinrichsen,, R. Lawson, V. Mountford, and K. Russell, *Cognitive Behavioral Therapy for Eating Disorders: A Comprehensive Treatment Guide* (New York: Cambridge University Press, 2007).

21. The figure of 200 calories per day is cited by K. K. Konrad, R. A. Carels, and D. M. Garner, "Metabolic and Psychological Changes during Refeeding in Anorexia Nervosa," *Eating & Weight Disorders* 12 (2007): 20–26. The 380-calorie-per-day figure is found in M. Marra, A. Polito, E. De Filippo, M. Cuzzolaro, D. Ciarapica, F. Contaldo, and L. Scalfi, "Are the General Equations to Predict BMR Applicable to Patients with Anorexia Nervosa?" *Eating & Weight Disorders* 7 (2002): 53–59.

22. V. Van Wymelbeke, L. Brondel, J. M. Brun, and D. Rigaud, "Factors Associated with the Increase in Resting Energy Expenditure during Refeeding in Malnourished Anorexia Nervosa Patients," *American Journal of Clinical Nutrition* 80 (2004): 1469–77.

23. J. E. Wildes and M. D. Marcus, "Weight Suppression as a Predictor of Weight Gain and Response to Intensive Behavioral Treatment in Patients with Anorexia Nervosa," *Behaviour Research and Therapy* 50 (2012): 266–74;

and F. A. Carter, V. V. McIntosh, P. R. Joyce, and C. M. Bulik, "Weight Suppression Predicts Weight Gain over Treatment but Not Treatment Completion or Outcome in Bulimia Nervosa," *Journal of Abnormal Psychology* 117 (2008): 936–40.

Chapter 8: Get Moving (or Not): What's Best for You?

1. "The Biggest Loser 601," *The Biggest Loser,* NBC. September 16, 2008.

2. Lululemon Athletica, "the lululemon manifesto," photograph 2012, *Lululemon.org,* www.lululemon.com/about/manifesto# (accessed September 2, 2012).

3. U.S. Department of Health and Human Services, *The Surgeon General's Vision for a Healthy and Fit Nation* (Rockville, MD: U.S. Department of Health and Human Services, Office of the Surgeon General, January 2010).

4. E. C. Adkins and P. K. Keel, "Does 'Excessive' or 'Compulsive' Best Describe Exercise as a Symptom of Bulimia Nervosa?" *International Journal of Eating Disorders* 38 (2005): 24–29; and C. Meyer and L. Taranis, "Exercise in the Eating Disorders: Terms and Definitions," *European Eating Disorders Review* 19 (2011): 169–73.

5. L. Taranis, S. Touyz, and C. Meyer, "Disordered Eating and Exercise: Development and Preliminary Validation of the Compulsive Exercise Test," *European Eating Disorders Review* 19 (2011): 256–68.

6. C. Boyd, S. Abraham, and G. Luscombe, "Exercise Behaviors and Feelings in Eating Disorder and Non-eating Disorder Groups," *European Eating Disorders Review* 15 (2007): 112–28.

7. S. Springer, "Defending Champion: How Geoffrey Mutai Trains for the Boston Marathon," *The Boston Globe,* April 13, 2012.

8. P. Friedman, *Diary of an Exercise Addict* (Guilford: Globe Pequot Press, 2009), 183–84.

9. H. Shroff, L. Reba, L. M. Thornton, F. Tozzi, K. L. Klump, W. H. Berrettini, H. Brandt, S. Crawford, S. Crow, M. M. Fichter, D. Goldman, K. A. Halmi, C. Johnson, A. S. Kaplan, P. Keel, M. LaVia, J. Mitchell, A. Rotondo, M. Strober, J. Treasure, D. B. Woodside, W. H. Kaye, and C. M. Bulik, "Features Associated with Excessive Exercise in Women with Eating Disorders," *International Journal of Eating Disorders* 39 (2006): 454–61; and C. Davis and S. Kaptein, "Anorexia Nervosa with Excessive Exercise: A Phenotype with Close Links to Obsessive-Compulsive Disorder," *Psychiatry Research* 142 (2006): 209–17.

10. Friedman, *Diary of an Exercise Addict,* 183–84.

11. M. Wilson, R. O'Hanlon, S. Prasad, A. Deighan, P. Macmillan, D. Oxborough, R. Godfrey, G. Smith, A. Maceira, S. Sharma, K. George, and G. Whyte, "Diverse Patterns of Myocardial Fibrosis in Lifelong, Veteran Endurance Athletes," *Journal of Applied Physiology* 110 (2011): 1622–26.

12. J. J. Thomas, P. K. Keel, and T. F. Heatherton, "Disordered Eating and Injuries among Adolescent Ballet Dancers," *Eating and Weight Disorders* 16 (2011): 215–22.

13. Dotsie Bausch (Cyclist), email message with Jenni Schaefer, October 8, 2012.

14. Shroff et al., "Features Associated with Excessive Exercise in Women with Eating Disorders."

15. J. Rimer, K. Dwan, D. A. Lawlor, C. A Greig, M. McMurdo, W. Morley, and G. E. Mead, "Exercise for Depression (Review)," *The Cochrane Library* 7 (2012).

16. E. J. Waugh, D. B. Woodside, D. E. Beaton, P. Cote, and G. A. Hawker, "Effects of Exercise on Bone Mass in Young Women with Anorexia Nervosa," *Medicine & Science in Sports & Exercise* 43 (2011): 755–63.

17. N. Hieber and M. E. Berrett, "Intuitive Exercise," *Center for Change*, October 2003, www.centerforchange.com/news-resources/newsletter/intuitive exercise (accessed December 4, 2012).

18. Beth Hartman McGilley (Clinical Psychologist), email message with Jenni Schaefer, October 16, 2012.

19. T. R. Carei, A. L. Fyfe-Johnson, C. C. Breuner, and M. A. Brown, "Randomized Controlled Clinical Trial of Yoga in the Treatment of Eating Disorders," *Journal of Adolescent Health* 46 (2010): 346–51.

20. J. J. Thomas, P. K. Keel, and T. F. Heatherton "Disordered Eating Attitudes and Behaviors in Ballet Students: Examination of Environmental and Individual Risk Factors," *International Journal of Eating Disorders* 38 (2005) 263–68.

21. R. C. Casper, E. L. Sullivan, and L. Tecott, "Relevance of Animal Models to Human Eating Disorders and Obesity," *Psychopharmacology* 199 (2008) 313–29.

Chapter 9: Accepting and Loving Your Body (Yes, We Said Loving!)

1. Bulik, *How to Stop Confusing What You Look Like with Who You Are*, 177–78.

2. R. H. Salk and R. E. Engeln-Maddox, "Fat Talk among College Women is Both Contagious and Harmful," *Sex Roles* 66 (2012): 636–45.

3. "Fat Talk Free Pledge," BodyImage3D, http://bi3d.tridelta.org/Pledge (accessed October 31, 2012).

4. L. Bloom, "How to Talk to Little Girls," *Huffington Post*, June 22, 2011, www.huffingtonpost.com/lisa-bloom/how-to-talk-to-little-gir_b_882510.html (accessed January 1, 2012).

5. Written by Jenni Schaefer, Teresa Boaz, and Sandy Ramos. © 2010 Hello Me Music (BMI)/Striper Music (BMI)/Lawyer's Wife Music (BMI)/Bodell Music (BMI). All rights reserved. International copyright secured. Used by permission.

6. L. Smolak and S. K. Murnen, "A Meta-analytic Examination of the Relationship between Child Sexual Abuse and Eating Disorders," *International Journal of Eating Disorders* 31 (2002) 136–50; and E. D. Konsky and A. Moyer, "Childhood Sexual Abuse and Non-suicidal Self-Injury: Meta-analysis," *British Journal of Psychiatry* 192 (2008): 166–70.

7. R. Shafran, M. Lee, E. Payne, and C. G. Fairburn, "An Experimental Analysis of Body Checking," *Behaviour Research and Therapy* 45 (2007) 113–21.

8. D. J. Simons and C. F. Chabris, "Gorillas in Our Midst: Sustained Inattentional Blindness for Dynamic Events," *Perception* 28 (1999) 1059–74.

9. D. T. Levin and D. J. Simons, "Failure to Detect Changes to Attended Objects in Motion Pictures," *Psychonomic Bulletin and Review* 4 (1997): 501–6.

10. Sherrie Delinsky (Clinical Psychologist), email message with Jennifer J. Thomas, November 29, 2012.

11. T. Hildebrandt, K. Loeb, S. Troupe, and S. Delinsky, "Adjunctive Mirror Exposure for Eating Disorders: A Randomized Controlled Pilot Study," *Behaviour Research and Therapy* 50 (2012): 797–804.

12. C. Boyle, *Operation Beautiful: Transforming the Way You See Yourself One Post-it Note at a Time* (New York: Penguin Group, 2010).

13. The Center for Eating Disorders at Sheppard Pratt, "Public Survey Conducted by the Center for Eating Disorders at Sheppard Pratt Finds Facebook Use Impacts the Way Many People Feel about Their Bodies." www.prnewswire.com/news-releases-test/public-survey-conducted-by-the-center-for-eating-disorders-at-sheppard-pratt-reveals-that-facebook-drains-body-image-and-self-esteem-144601505.html

14. T. M. Leahey, J. H. Crowther, and J. A. Ciesla, "An Ecological Momentary Assessment of the Effects of Weight and Shape Social Comparisons on Women with Eating Pathology, High Body Dissatisfaction, and Low Body Dissatisfaction," *Behavior Therapy* 42 (2011) 197–210.

15. J. Weiner, *Life Doesn't Begin 5 Pounds from Now* (New York: Simon & Schuster, 2007).

16. K. Harding, "The Fantasy of Being Thin," *Shapely Prose*, November 27, 2007, kateharding.net/2007/11/27/the-fantasy-of-being-thin (accessed October 31, 2012).

17. Written by Jenni Schaefer, Dave Berg, and Georgia Middleman. © 2009 Hello Me Music (BMI)/Cal IV Songs (ASCAP)/Stupid Boy Music (ASCAP)/Middle Girl Music (ASCAP). All rights reserved. International copyright secured. Used by permission. All rights on behalf of Cal IV Songs and Stupid Boy Music administered by Cal IV Entertainment, LLC, 808 19th Avenue South, Nashville, TN 37203.

18. A. Liddon, "Size Healthy Contest," Oh She Glows, February 17, 2010, http://ohsheglows.com/2010/02/17/size-healthy-contest/ (accessed October 31, 2012).

19. P. K. Keel, D. J. Dorer, D. L. Franko, S. C. Jackson, and D. B. Herzog, "Postremission Predictors of Relapse in Women with Eating Disorders," *American Journal of Psychiatry* 162 (2005): 2263–68.

Chapter 10: It's Not Just You and Ed: Creating a Circle of Support

1. I. Krug, E. Penelo, F. Fernandez-Aranda, M. Anderluh, L. Bellodi, E. Cellini, M. di Bernando, R. Granero, A. Karwautz, B. Nacmias, V. Ricca, S. Sorbi, K. Tchanturia, G. Wagner, D. Collier, and J. Treasure, "Low Social Interactions in Eating Disorder Patients in Childhood and Adulthood: A Multi-centre European Case Control Study," *Journal of Health Psychology*, in press.

2. A. Wright and M. E. Pritchard, "An Examination of the Relation of Gender, Mass Media Influence, and Loneliness to Disordered Eating among College Students," *Eating and Weight Disorders* 14 (2009): e144–47.

3. C. A. Levinson and T. L. Rodebaugh, "Social Anxiety and Eating Disorder Comorbidity: The Role of Negative Social Evaluation Fears," *Eating Behaviors* 13 (2012): 27–35; and D. M. Hamann, A. L. Wonderlich-Tierney, and J. S. Vander, "Interpersonal Sensitivity Predicts Bulimic Symptomatology Cross-Sectionally and Longitudinally," *Eating Behaviors* 10 (2009) 125–27.

4. T. D. Wade, S. M. Wilksch, and C. Lee, "A Longitudinal Investigation of the Impact of Disordered Eating on Young Women's Quality of Life," *Health Psychology* 31 (2012): 352–59.

5. F. M. Cachelin and R. H. Striegel-Moore, "Help Seeking and Barriers to Treatment in a Community Sample of Mexican American and European American Women with Eating Disorders," *International Journal of Eating Disorders* 39 (2006): 154–61; and A. E. Becker, A. H. Arrindell, A. Perloe, K. Fay, and R. H. Striegel-Moore, "A Qualitative Study of Perceived Social Barriers to Care for Eating Disorders: Perspectives from Ethnically Diverse Health Care Consumers," *International Journal of Eating Disorders* 43 (2010): 633–47.

6. Cachelin and Striegel-Moore, "Help Seeking and Barriers to Treatment in a Community Sample of Mexican American and European American Women with Eating Disorders."

7. G. Pettersen, J. H. Rosenvinge, and B. Ytterhus, "The 'Double Life' of Bulimia: Patients' Experiences in Daily Life Interactions," *Eating Disorders* 16 (2008): 204–11.

8. "Prescott Tells of Bulimia Battle," *BBC News*, April 20, 2008, at news.bbc .co.uk/2/hi/uk_politics/7357008.stm (accessed November 5, 2012).

9. Cachelin and Striegel-Moore, "Help Seeking and Barriers to Treatment in a Community Sample of Mexican American and European American Women with Eating Disorders."

10. A. E. Becker, J. J. Thomas, D. L. Franko, and D. B. Herzog, "Disclosure Patterns of Eating and Weight Concerns to Clinicians, Educational Professionals, Family, and Peers," *International Journal of Eating Disorders* 38 (2005): 18–23.

11. P. S. Richards, R. K. Hardman, and M. E. Berrett, *Spiritual Approaches in the Treatment of Women With Eating Disorders* (USA: American Psychological Association, 2006).

12. M.E. Berrett, N. Button, and P. Levine, "Spirituality and Religion in Eating Disorder Development, Treatment and Recovery" (presentation at the National Eating Disorders Association Conference, St. Petersburg, Florida, October 2012).

13. P. S. Richards, M. E. Berret, R. K. Hardman, and D. L. Eggett, "Comparative Efficacy of Spirituality, Cognitive, and Emotional Support Groups for Treating Eating Disorder Inpatients," *Eating Disorders* 14 (2006): 401–15.

14. M. E. Berrett, "Reciprocal Social Support of Adolescents: An Assessment Model and Measure" (PhD dissertation, Brigham Young University, 1985).

15. P. K. Keel, K. J. Forney, T. A. Brown, and T. F. Heatherton, "Influence of College Peers on Disordered Eating in Women and Men at 10-Year Follow-Up," *Journal of Abnormal Psychology*, in press (2012).

16. C. G. Fairburn, Z. Cooper, H. A. Doll, M. E. O'Connor, K. Bohn, D. M. Hawker, J. A. Wales, and R. L. Palmer, "Transdiagnostic Cognitive-Behavioral Therapy for Patients with Eating Disorders: A Two-Site Trial with 60-Week Follow-Up," *American Journal of Psychiatry* 166 (2009): 311–19.

17. J. Lock, D. Le Grange, W. S. Agras, A. Moye, S. W. Bryson, and B. Jo, "Randomized Clinical Trial Comparing Family-Based Treatment with Adolescent-Focused Individual Therapy for Adolescents with Anorexia Nervosa," *Archives of General Psychiatry* 67 (2010): 1025–32.

18. C. M. Bulik, D. H. Baucom, J. S. Kirby, and E. Pisetsky, "Uniting Couples (in the Treatment of) Anorexia Nervosa (UCAN)," *International Journal of Eating Disorders* 44 (2011): 19–28.

19. S. J. Romano, K. A. Halmi, N. P. Sarkar, S. C. Koke, and J. S. Lee, "A Placebo-Controlled Study of Fluoxetine in Continued Treatment of Bulimia Nervosa after Successful Acute Fluoxetine Treatment," *American Journal of Psychiatry* 159 (2002): 96–102.

20. H. Bissada, G. A. Tasca, A. M. Barber, and J. Bradwejn, "Olanzapine in the Treatment of Low Body Weight and Obsessive Thinking in Women with Anorexia Nervosa: A Randomized, Double-Blind, Placebo-Controlled Trial," *American Journal of* Psychiatry 165 (2008): 1281–88.

21. S. L. McElroy, J. I. Hudson, J. A. Capece, K. Beyers, A. C. Fisher, N. R. Rosenthal, and Topiramate Binge Eating Disorder Research Group, "Topiramate for the Treatment of Binge Eating Disorder Associated with Obesity: A Placebo-Controlled Study," *Biological Psychiatry* 61 (2007): 1039–48.

22. R. L. Horne, J. M. Ferguson, H. G. Pope Jr., J. I. Hudson, C. G. Lineberry, J. Ascher, and A. Cato, "Treatment of Bulimia with Bupropion: A Multicenter Controlled Trial," *Journal of Clinical Psychology* 49 (1998) 262–66.

23. American Psychiatric Association, "Treatment of Patients with Eating Disorders," *American Journal of Psychiatry* 163 (2006): 4–54.

24. K. M. Von Ranson, S. K. Russell-Mayhew, and P. C. Masson, "An Exploratory Study of Eating Disorder Psychopathology among Overeaters Anonymous Members," *Eating and Weight Disorders* 16 (2011): e65–68.

25. J. Treasure, G. Smith, and A. Crane, *Skills-Based Learning for Caring for a Loved One with an Eating Disorder: The New Maudsley Method* (New York: Routledge, 2007).

26. S. Cutts, *Beating Ana: How to Outsmart Your Eating Disorder and Take Your Life Back* (Deerfield Beach, FL: Health Communications Inc., 2009), 7.

Chapter 11: Don't Settle for Almost Recovered

1. K. T. Eddy, S. A. Swanson, R. D. Crosby, D. L. Franko, S. Engel, and D. B. Herzog, "How Should DSM-V Classify Eating Disorder Not Otherwise Specified (EDNOS) Presentations in Women with Lifetime Anorexia or Bulimia Nervosa?" *Psychological Medicine* 40 (2010): 1735–44.

2. C. Costin, *100 Questions & Answers about Eating Disorders* (Boston: Jones and Bartlett Publishers, 2007), 164.

3. A. M. Darcy, S. Katz, K. K. Fitzpatrick, S. Forsberg, L. Utzinger, and J. Lock, "All Better? How Former Anorexia Nervosa Patients Define Recovery and Engaged in Treatment," *European Eating Disorders Review* 18 (2010): 260–70.

4. U. Schmidt, S. Lee, S. Perkins, I. Eisler, J. Treasure, J. Beecham, M. Berelowitz, L. Dodge, S. Frost, M. Jenkins, E. Johnson-Sabine, S. Keville, R. Murphey, P. Robinson, S. Winn, and I. Yi, "Do Adolescents with Eating Disorder Not Otherwise Specified or Full-Syndrome Bulimia Nervosa Differ in Clinical Severity, Comorbidity, Risk Factors, Treatment Outcome or Cost?," *International Journal of Eating Disorders* 41 (2008): 498–504; L. Nevonen and A. G. Broberg, "A Comparison of Sequenced Individual and Group Psychotherapy for Eating Disorder Not Otherwise Specified," *European Eating Disorders Review* 13 (2005): 29–37; C. G. Fairburn, Z. Cooper, H. A. Doll, M. E. O'Connor, K. Bohn, D. M. Hawker, J. A. Wales, and R. L. Palmer, "Transdiagnostic Cognitive-Behavioral Therapy for Patients with Eating Disorders: A Two-Site Trial with 60-Week Follow-Up," *American Journal of Psychiatry* 166 (2009): 311–19.

5. W. S. Agras, S. Crow, J. E. Mitchell, K. A. Halmi, and S. Bryson, "A 4-Year Prospective Study of Eating Disorder NOS Compared with Full Eating Disorder Syndromes," *International Journal of Eating Disorders* 42 (2009): 565–70; and C. M. Grilo, M. E. Pagano, A. E. Skodol, C. A. Sanislow, T. H. McGlashan, J. G. Gunderson, and R. L. Stout, "Natural Course of

Bulimia Nervosa and of Eating Disorder Not Otherwise Specified: 5-Year Prospective Study of Remissions, Relapses, and the Effects of Personality Disorder Psychopathology," *Journal of Clinical Psychiatry* 68 (2007): 738–46.

6. Lock, Le Grange, Agras, and Dare, *Treatment Manual for Anorexia Nervosa: A Family-Based Approach*; and Fairburn, *Cognitive Behavior Therapy and Eating Disorders*.

7. D. Le Grange and J. Lock, "The Dearth of Psychological Treatment Studies for Anorexia Nervosa," *International Journal of Eating Disorders* 37 (2005): 79–91.

8. Fairburn, Cooper, Doll, O'Connor, Bohn, Hawker, Wales, and Palmer, "Transdiagnostic Cognitive-Behavioral Therapy for Patients with Eating Disorders: A Two-Site Trial with 60-Week Follow-Up."

9. Keel, Dorer, Franko, Jackson, and Herzog, "Postremission Predictors of Relapse in Women with Eating Disorders"; J. Schebendach, L. Mayer, M. J. Devlin, E. Attia, and B. T, Walsh, "Dietary Energy Density and Diet Variety in Anorexia Nervosa: A Replication," *International Journal of Eating Disorders* 45 (2012): 79–84; and J. C. Carter, E. Blackmore, K. Sutandar-Pinnock, and D. B. Woodside, "Relapse in Anorexia Nervosa: A Survival Analysis," *Psychological Medicine* 34 (2004): 671–79.

10. G. M. Grilo, M. E. Pagano, R. L. Stout, J. C. Markowitz, E. B. Ansell, A. Pinto, M. C. Zanarini, S. Yen, A. E. Skodol, "Stressful Life Events Predict Eating Disorder Relapse Following Remission: Six-Year Prospective Outcomes," *International Journal of Eating Disorders* 45 (2012): 185–92; and Keel, Dorer, Franko, Jackson, and Herzog, "Postremission Predictors of Relapse in Women with Eating Disorders."

11. J. M. Holm-Denoma, K. D. Vohs, and T. F. Heatherton, "The 'Freshman Fifteen' (the 'Freshman Five' Actually): Predictors and Possible Explanations," *Health Psychology* 27 (2008): S3–9.

12. D. L. Cohen and T. A. Petri, "An Examination of Psychosocial Correlates of Disordered Eating among Undergraduate Women," *Sex Roles* 52 (2005): 29–42.

13. J. M. Lavender, K. P. De Young, and D. A. Anderson "Eating Disorder Examination Questionnaire (EDE-Q): Norms for Undergraduate Men," *Eating Behaviors* 11 (2010): 119–21.

14. Margo Maine (Clinical Psychologist), email message with Jenni Schaefer, October 22, 2012.

15. Reba Sloan (Dietitian), email message with Jenni Schaefer, November 4, 2012.

16. Kamryn Eddy (Clinical Psychologist), email message with Jennifer J. Thomas, October 6, 2012.

17. Amanda Olsen (Eating Disorder Survivor), email message with Jenni Schaefer, August 28, 2012.

18. Mark Warren (Physician), email message with Jenni Schaefer, November 15, 2012.

19. A. Keski-Rahkonen and F. Tozzi, "The Process of Recovery in Eating Disorder Sufferers' Own Words: An Internet-Based Study," *International Journal of Eating Disorders*, 37 (2005): S80–86.

permissions

Chapter 1

The EAT-26 has been reproduced with permission. Garner et al., "The Eating Attitudes Test: Psychometric Features and Clinical Correlates," *Psychological Medicine* 12 (1982), 871–78.

Chapter 8

The Compulsive Exercise Test has been reproduced with permission. Loren Taranis, Stephen Touyz, and Caroline Meyer, "Compulsive Exercise Test," *European Eating Disorders Review*, 19:3 (2011), 256–68.

Chapter 9

The Fat Talk Free® Pledge is the property of Delta Delta Delta sorority. Used with permission.

Lyrics for "She Blames Herself" are written by Jenni Schaefer, Teresa Boaz, and Sandy Ramos. © 2010 Hello Me Music (BMI)/Striper Music (BMI)/Lawyer's Wife Music (BMI)/Cauley Music Group (BMI). All rights reserved. International copyright secured. Used by permission.

Lyrics for "It's Okay to Be Happy" are written by Jenni Schaefer, Dave Berg, and Georgia Middleman. © 2009 Hello Me Music (BMI)/Cal IV Songs (ASCAP)/Stupid Boy Music (ASCAP)/Middle Girl Music (ASCAP). All rights reserved. International copyright secured. Used by permission. All rights on behalf of Cal IV Songs and Stupid Boy Music, administered by Cal IV Entertainment, LLC, 808 19th Avenue South, Nashville, TN 37203.

about the authors

Dr. Jennifer Thomas is assistant professor of psychology at Harvard Medical School and assistant director of the Eating Disorders Clinical and Research Program at Massachusetts General Hospital. Her groundbreaking scientific research, which focuses on the development of an eating disorder typology that better reflects clinical reality, has been funded by the National Institute of Mental Health, the Klarman Family Foundation, and the Hilda and Preston Davis Foundation. She has published forty scientific articles and chapters, serves on the editorial boards of *International Journal of Eating Disorders* and *Journal of Abnormal Psychology*, and is a member of the Academy for Eating Disorders and Eating Disorders Research Society. She lives in downtown Boston, where she also maintains a private psychotherapy practice, helping people with almost anorexia and other officially recognized eating disorders. Connect with her online at www.jennifer jthomasphd.com.

Jenni Schaefer's breakthrough bestseller, *Life Without Ed: How One Woman Declared Independence from Her Eating Disorder and How You Can Too*, established her as one of the leading lights in the recovery movement. With her second book, *Goodbye Ed, Hello Me: Recover from Your Eating Disorder and Fall in Love with Life*, she earned her place as one of the country's foremost motivational writers and speakers. Jenni's straightforward, realistic style has made her a role model, source of inspiration, and confidant to people worldwide looking to overcome adversity and live more fully. She speaks at conferences, at

315

major universities, and in corporate settings; has appeared on many syndicated TV and radio shows; and has been quoted in publications including *The New York Times*. She is also chair of the Ambassadors Council of the National Eating Disorders Association. An accomplished singer/songwriter, she lives in Austin, Texas. For more information or to contact Jenni, visit www.jennischaefer.com.

Hazelden, a national nonprofit organization founded in 1949, helps people reclaim their lives from the disease of addiction. Built on decades of knowledge and experience, Hazelden offers a comprehensive approach to addiction that addresses the full range of patient, family, and professional needs, including treatment and continuing care for youth and adults, research, higher learning, public education and advocacy, and publishing.

A life of recovery is lived "one day at a time." Hazelden publications, both educational and inspirational, support and strengthen lifelong recovery. In 1954, Hazelden published *Twenty-Four Hours a Day*, the first daily meditation book for recovering alcoholics, and Hazelden continues to publish works to inspire and guide individuals in treatment and recovery, and their loved ones. Professionals who work to prevent and treat addiction also turn to Hazelden for evidence-based curricula, informational materials, and videos for use in schools, treatment programs, and correctional programs.

Through published works, Hazelden extends the reach of hope, encouragement, help, and support to individuals, families, and communities affected by addiction and related issues.

For questions about Hazelden publications, please call **800-328-9000** or visit us online at **hazelden.org/bookstore.**